A practical handbook on the pharmacovigilance of antimalarial medicines

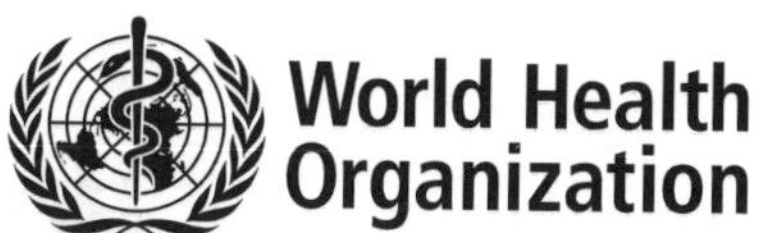

WHO Library Cataloguing-in-Publication Data

A practical handbook on the pharmacovigilance of antimalarial medicines.

1.Drug monitoring. 2.Antimalarials - adverse effects. 3.Adverse drug reaction reporting systems. 4.Drug utilization review - methods. I.World Health Organization.

ISBN 978 92 4 154749 9 (NLM classification: QV 771)

Printed by WHO Document Production Services, Geneva, Switzerland

Acknowledgements

This publication was developed following two training courses in Zambia and Ghana in 2007. The manuscript was drafted by David Coulter who was responsible for the Intensive Medicines Monitoring Programme in New Zealand and sincere thanks are expressed to him for his dedication. The draft was reviewed by members of the Advisory Committee on the Safety of Medicinal Products.

Art Direction: Jean-Claude Fattier, WHO

Photograph design: Caroline Scudamore, WHO

WHO expresses its sincere appreciation to the European Community for providing financial support to the development of this publication.

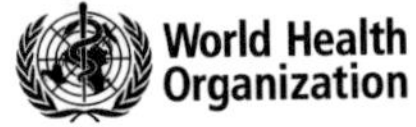

A practical handbook on the pharmacovigilance of antimalarial medicines

A practical handbook on the pharmacovigilance of antimalarial medicines

A. Introduction

This is a detailed manual giving a step by step approach to undertaking the pharmacovigilance of antimalarials. It is intended to be a source of practical advice for Pharmacovigilance Centres. A number of WHO publications are available that provide a background to pharmacovigilance and, as far as possible, that material will not be repeated here. Health officials, planners, the staff of Pharmacovigilance Centres and all health workers should become familiar with these publications, which are:

- *Safety of medicines: A guide to detecting and reporting adverse drug reactions*
- *The importance of pharmacovigilance: safety monitoring of medicinal products*
- *Safety monitoring of medicinal products: guidelines for setting up and running a Pharmacovigilance Centre*
- *The safety of medicines in public health programmes: pharmacovigilance an essential tool*

These booklets are available free from Quality Assurance and Safety of Medicines, WHO, Geneva, Switzerland.

1. Pharmacovigilance

Definition

Pharmacovigilance has been defined as: *The science and activities relating to the detection, assessment, understanding and prevention of adverse effects or any other drug-related problem* (WHO).

Explanation

Pharmacovigilance is an arm of patient care. It aims at getting the best outcome of treatment with medicines. No one wants to harm patients, but unfortunately, because of many different factors, any medicine will sometimes do this. Good pharmacovigilance will identify the risks in the shortest possible time after the medicine has been marketed and will help to establish/identify risk factors. When communicated effectively, this information allows for intelligent, evidence-based prescribing with potential for preventing many adverse reactions and will ultimately help each patient to receive optimum therapy at a lower cost to the health system.

Pharmacovigilance of antimalarials

Malaria is the greatest killer disease of all time. Unfortunately, after a period of relatively good control in many countries with the use of insecticides and antimalarials such as chloroquine, there has been a resurgence of this disease. This is due to the development of resistance of mosquitoes to insecticides and resistance of parasites to the antimalarials, thus producing an increase in malaria morbidity and mortality. WHO is promoting the use of artemisinin combination therapies (ACTs) as a therapeutic tool to treat uncomplicated acute falciparum malaria. It is known to be effective, but its safety under large-scale operational use has not been fully assessed. Children and pregnant women are the most vulnerable to falciparum malaria and least is known about safety in these populations. A range of ACTs is becoming available and it is important that these are carefully monitored.

2. Pharmacovigilance centre

The Pharmacovigilance Centre is responsible for meeting the requirements for good pharmacovigilance of all medicines and is a centre of expertise for the art and science of monitoring and analysis and the use of the analysed information for the benefit of patients. National and any regional Pharmacovigilance Centres should be set up with the approval of the authority responsible for the regulation of medicines ("regulatory authority"). The centre may function within the regulatory authority, a hospital, an academic institution or as an independent facility such as a trust or foundation.

B. Passive or active pharmacovigilance?

1. Passive pharmacovigilance

Passive surveillance means that no active measures are taken to look for adverse effects other than the encouragement of health professionals and others to report safety concerns. Reporting is entirely dependent on the initiative and motivation of the potential reporters. This is the most common form of pharmacovigilance. It is commonly referred to as "spontaneous" or "voluntary" reporting. In some countries this form of reporting is mandatory.

2. Active pharmacovigilance

Active (or proactive) safety surveillance means that active measures are taken to detect adverse events. This is managed by active follow-up after treatment and the events may be detected by asking patients directly or screening patient records. It is best done prospectively. Active pharmacovigilance is sometimes very descriptively referred to as, "hot pursuit". The most comprehensive method is cohort event monitoring (CEM). Examples of this are the Intensive Medicines Monitoring Programme (IMMP) in New Zealand and Prescription Event Monitoring (PEM) in England. Other methods used include the use of registers, record linkage and screening of laboratory results in medical laboratories.

Methods for both passive (spontaneous reporting) and active pharmacovigilance (CEM) will be described. The essential and interesting tasks of causality assessment and signal identification are applicable to both methods of surveillance and will be covered in detail after the individual methods have been discussed.

C. Spontaneous reporting

1. Introduction

1.1. Background

1.1.1. A spontaneous report is an unsolicited communication by healthcare professionals or consumers that describes one or more adverse drug reactions in a patient who was given one or more medicinal products and that does not derive from a study or any organized data collection scheme.

1.1.2. Throughout the world spontaneous reporting is the most common method of surveillance. It is the easiest to establish and the cheapest to run, but reporting rates are generally very low and subject to strong biases and there is no database of all users or information on overall drug utilization. These problems prevent the accurate assessment of risk, risk factors or comparisons between drugs. Nevertheless spontaneous reporting has played a major role in the identification of safety signals throughout the marketed lifetime of medicines in general.

1.2 Adverse reactions

1.2.1 It should be noted that this method is for the reporting of suspected *adverse reactions*.

1.2.2. The definition of an adverse reaction is: *a response to a medicine which is noxious and unintended, and which occurs at doses normally used in man.* (WHO).

2. Objectives

2.1. The aims of spontaneous reporting are to:

2.1.1. improve patient care and safety in relation to the use of medicines and all medical and paramedical interventions;

2.1.2. improve public health and safety in relation to the use of medicines;

2.1.3. detect problems related to the use of medicines and communicate the findings in a timely manner;

2.1.4. contribute to the assessment of benefit, harm, effectiveness and risk of medicines, leading to the prevention of harm and maximization of benefit;

2.1.5. encourage the safe, rational and more effective (including cost-effective) use of medicines; and

2.1.6. promote understanding, education and clinical training in pharmacovigilance and its effective communication to the public.

2.2. Pharmacovigilance using a spontaneous reporting system is designed to detect adverse reactions not previously observed in preclinical or clinical studies, improve understanding of the potential risks, including reactions resulting from drug interactions or drug effects in particular populations, and to help provide a basis for effective drug regulation, education and consequent changes in practices by prescribers and consumers.

2.3. Spontaneous reporting in malarious countries has as a focus, population-based monitoring in order to detect, assess, communicate and respond to suspected *serious* adverse reactions.

2.3.1. *A **serious adverse reaction** is any untoward medical occurrence that at any dose results in death, is life threatening, requires or prolongs patient hospitalisation, results in persistent disability/incapacity, or is a congenital anomaly/birth defect* (International Conference on Harmonisation (ICH)).

2.3.2. The term "life-threatening" in the definition of "serious" refers to an event in which the patient was at risk of death at the time of the event; it does not refer to an event, which hypothetically might have caused death if it was more severe.

2.4. Summary of objectives

2.4.1. The identification of signals of serious adverse drug reactions following the introduction of a new drug or drug combination;

2.4.2. Assessment of signals to evaluate causality, clinical relevance, frequency and distribution in particular population groups;

2.4.3. Communications and recommendations to authorities and the public;

2.4.4. Appropriate response/action in terms of drug registration, drug use and/or training and education for health professionals and the public;

2.4.5. Measurement of outcome of response or of action taken (e.g. reduction in risk, improved drug use, or improved outcome for patients experiencing a detected adverse reaction).

2.5. Medical and scientific judgement should be exercised in deciding whether other situations are serious, such as important medical events that may not be immediately life threatening or result in death or hospitalization but may jeopardize the patient or may require intervention to prevent one of the outcomes listed in the definition above. Examples include blood dyscrasias or convulsions not resulting in hospitalization, or development of drug dependency or drug abuse.

3. Minimum reporting requirements

3.1. According to WHO criteria, the following basic information is required before a report is acceptable:

3.1.1 an identifiable source of information or reporter;

3.1.2. an identifiable patient;

3.1.3. name(s) of the suspected product(s);

3.1.4. a description of the suspected reaction(s).

3.2. The reporter must be literate

3.2.1. The system depends on written records using a standard reporting form. For this reason, the reporting system extends only to the clinic and dispensary level of the health care system.

3.2.2. Informal health care providers, because of their varying degrees of literacy, cannot act as reporters, but should play an important role in referring patients to health facilities to report reactions.

4. How to report

4.1. Reporting form

Over 100 different reporting forms are available. These have been individually developed by each country that has set up a Pharmacovigilance Centre. To be effective a reporting form needs to be available in the local language and have features relating it to the responsible authority e.g. a logo, and the address and contact details of the issuing institution.

4.1.1. Pharmacovigilance centres will have developed their own national reporting forms.

4.1.2. Forms should be simple and easy to complete.

4.1.3. They should not request too much information, particularly information that is difficult to find and record, or information that is unlikely to be used.

4.1.4. There should be sufficient space in which to describe the suspected reaction(s).

4.1.5. They should be widely distributed to all health professionals including those who are treating malaria and those who are working privately. Difficulty in finding a reporting form is a barrier to reporting.

4.1.6. The forms should be printed on a single page and easily folded and sealed. The return address should be printed on the outside, with postage pre-paid if forms are to be posted.

4.1.7. It is desirable to have only one type of reporting form available in the country for use for all medicines including anti-malarials.

4.2. Other options for reporting

Reporting needs to be made as convenient as possible. If other methods are available, they may be preferred by some health professionals. Preferences may vary between clinics and hospitals, private or government facilities and public health programmes. Suitable methods might include:

4.2.1. *Telephone*. The person receiving the report should have a reporting form to record the details and make sure that essential data is not missing.

4.2.2. *E-mail*. A written case report submitted by e-mail may be acceptable. Further details can be obtained by follow-up. Reporting forms can be sent to reporters as e-mail attachments and faxed or mailed to the Pharmacovigilance Centre when completed.

4.2.3. *Fax*. Sending reports by fax is equivalent to mailing the report, but faster. A fax machine is a very important asset for a national Pharmacovigilance Centre and its major sentinel sites.

4.2.4. *The Internet*. An Internet site is a valuable asset for a Pharmacovigilance Centre and a reporting form could be made available for downloading or for completion online (entering data through web-based data entry) if the site is secure.

5. Where to report

5.1. Reports should be sent to the Pharmacovigilance Centre.

5.2. If it is not practical to send the forms directly to the centre, it may be necessary to arrange points of collection at other sites as e.g. specific hospitals or clinics.

5.3. They should be stored securely to maintain confidentiality.

6. What to report

6.1. Essential data elements

6.1.1. *Patient details*

6.1.1.1. Health number: this may be a national identifier (preferred), hospital, clinic or study number.

6.1.1.2. Name: full name as an accurate identifier for follow-up purposes and avoidance of duplication.

6.1.1.3. Address: to allow for follow-up and accurate identification.

6.1.1.4.Sex.

6.1.1.5. Date of birth (preferred) or age (add 'est' if age is estimated).

6.1.1.6. Weight and height.

6.1.2. *Patient medical history of significance – examples*

6.1.2.1. Renal disease.

6.1.2.2. Liver disease.

6.1.2.3. AIDS.

6.1.2.4. Tuberculosis.

6.1.3. *Details of medicines*

6.1.3.1. Name(s): (this may be brand or generic) and formulation (e.g. tablets, syrup, injection). Brand name is preferred.

6.1.3.2. Mode of administration (e.g. oral, rectal, injection).

6.1.3.3. Indication(s) for use.

6.1.3.4. Dose: e.g. for antimalarials, treatment regimen prescribed; for other medicines, total daily dose.

6.1.3.5. Date of commencement.

6.1.3.6. Date of withdrawal.

6.1.3.7 Duration of use, if dates of commencement and withdrawal are not available.

6.1.3.8. All medicines being taken at the time of the event should be listed. Each suspect medicine can be indicated by an asterisk.

6.1.4. *Reaction details*

6.1.4.1. Date of onset.

6.1.4.2. Reporters should be asked to give a brief clinical description. They should not be asked to give the official pharmacovigilance reaction term.

6.1.4.3. Laboratory test results if available.

6.1.4.4. Outcome of event: full recovery, recovering, no change, permanent damage, worsening, death (with date).

6.1.4.5. Effect of rechallenge[1] (if any).

6.1.5. *Reporter details*

6.1.5.1. Name.

6.1.5.2. Contact details.

6.1.5.3. Status: e.g. physician, nurse, patient.

6.1.6. *Date of report*

6.2. Advice to reporters

6.2.1. Suggest that they report any adverse event of concern.

6.2.2. Report all suspected serious reactions. A serious reaction:

6.2.2.1. results in death;

6.2.2.2. is life-threatening;

6.2.2.3. requires hospitalization or prolongation of hospitalization;

6.2.2.4. results in persistent disability;

1 Rechallenge is the voluntary or inadvertant re-administration of a medicine suspected of causing an adverse reaction.

6.2.2.5. is a congenital defect.

6.2.3. Advise that they do not need to be sure that the medicine caused the event.

6.3. Follow-up when necessary

6.3.1. All reports of serious events should be followed up if details are incomplete. This may require the involvement of health professionals trained and appointed for this type of work.

6.3.2. Occasionally follow-up information is required to fully assess reports of non-serius events. Follow-up requests should be kept to a minimum because they can act as a deterrent to further reporting. Examples might be:

6.3.2.1. a request for essential missing details;

6.3.2.2. information on the final outcome;

6.3.2.3. the result of rechallenge;

6.3.2.4. the results of laboratory tests;

6.3.2.5. postmortem results, from health facilities where autopsy is undertaken.

7. When to report

7.1. A report should be completed as soon as possible after the reaction.

7.2. It is better to advise reporters not to wait until final results and information such as hospital letters are received, because the report may be forgotten. These additional details can be sent to the Pharmacovigilance Centre later.

8. Who should report

The following is a list of potential reporters. They may work in the public or private health sectors.

8.1. Physicians.

8.2. Pharmacists.

8.3. Nurses.

8.4. Other (literate) health workers.

8.5. Public health programmes.

8.6. Pharmaceutical companies.

8.7. Patients or patient representatives.

9. Sharing the results

9.1. Individual, immediate

9.1.1. Anyone who sends in a report should receive a letter of thanks and further reporting forms.

9.1.2. In addition, the letter should provide some *brief* information about the reaction reported, such as, but not normally including all, of the following:

9.1.2.1. number of reports of the reaction in the centre's database;

9.1.2.2. number of reports of the reaction in the WHO database;

9.1.2.3. information from the literature;

9.1.2.4. the importance of the reaction in the management of malaria cases;

9.1.2.5. the safety or risk of further administration to the patient;

9.1.2.6. the possibility of preventing the reaction in other patients by indicating potential risk factors.

9.2. Relevant summaries or reviews

9.2.1. From time to time, the Centre should prepare a summary of the reactions reported and/or safety reviews of the antimalarials being used locally.

9.2.2. These should be distributed widely as bulletins or newsletters.

9.2.3. News items should be prepared for the local media on overall effectiveness and safety, or about particular issues that have arisen.

9.3. Regular transmission to the WHO database

Details of reports should be sent to the WHO Collaborating Centre for International Drug Monitoring (the Uppsala Monitoring Centre) for inclusion in the worldwide database of the WHO Collaborating Programme on the safety of medicines The use of VigiFlow (described below) simplifies this procedure.

10. Data entry

10.1. Options

There are few, if any, commercial software products available to suit the needs of Pharmacovigilance Centres for data entry, storage and analysis. The UMC can provide access to VigiFlow which is a tool designed for these functions. It is the best option available.

10.2. VigiFlow

10.2.1. It is web based and requires no local support or maintenance.

10.2.2. It provides for standardized entry of data from reports.

10.2.3. It has built-in error avoidance features.

10.2.4. It provides access to a search and statistics database online.

10.2.5. National data can be accessed and used only by the local Pharmacovigilance Centre.

10.2.6. Standardized outputs are available for:

10.2.6.1. summary tabulations;

10.2.6.2. a range of standard statistical analyses.

10.2.7. The data can be exported to a local internal database for ad hoc searches and to meet local analytical requirements.

10.2.8. It provides live access to up-to-date terminologies:

10.2.8.1. WHO Drug Dictionary (DD).

10.2.8.2. WHO Adverse Reactions Terminology (WHO-ART).

10.2.9. The completed reports can be easily exported to the WHO database.

D. Cohort event monitoring

1. Introduction

1.1. Event monitoring

1.1.1. Definition

1.1.1.1. An adverse event (sometimes called an adverse experience) is defined as, "Any untoward medical occurrence temporally associated (i.e. associated in time) with the use of a medicinal product, but not necessarily causally related" (WHO).

1.1.1.2. Explanation

An event is any new clinical experience that occurs after commencing a medicine regardless of its severity or seriousness and without judgement on its causality. (Favourable events may be recorded as an indication of an unexpected therapeutic effect.)

1.1.1.3. Cohort Event Monitoring (CEM) records all clinical events and not just suspected adverse reactions.

1.1.2. Event monitoring involves

1.1.2.1. actively asking for reports of the events

1.1.2.2. systematically asking for reports of the events.

1.2. Description

1.2.1. Cohort event monitoring (CEM) is a prospective, observational, cohort study of adverse *events* associated with in one or more medicines.

1.2.2. This methodology is often referred to as prescription event monitoring (PEM), but this terminology is inappropriate when individual prescriptions with subsequent dispensing by pharmacists are not part of the process of supplying medicines to patients. In most malaria-endemic countries, the treatment of malaria is not provided on a prescription basis. Examples of CEM methodology are the Intensive Medicines Monitoring Programme (IMMP) in New Zealand and the PEM run by the

Drug Safety Research Unit in England.

1.2.3. A CEM programme is essentially an observational study of a new medicine in the early postmarketing phase, but it can be used for older medicines.

1.2.4. Its basic function is to act as an *early warning system* of problems with new medicines, although it will provide much more.

1.3. Objectives

1.3.1. The objectives of spontaneous reporting (see section C.2) are also objectives of CEM. The aims of CEM include the following, either in addition, or more effectively than for spontaneous reporting.

1.3.2. Provide incidence rates for adverse events as a measure of risk.

1.3.3. Characterize known adverse reactions.

1.3.4. Detect signals of unrecognized reactions.

1.3.5. Detect interactions with other medicines, complementary and alternative medicines, foods and concomitant diseases.

1.3.6. Identify risk factors and thus provide evidence on which to base effective risk management.

1.3.7. Assess safety in pregnancy and lactation.

1.3.8. Provide a measure of comparative risks between medicines.

1.3.9. Provide cohorts for further study of safety issues if required in the future.

1.3.10. Detect inefficacy, which might be due to:

1.3.10.1. faulty administration;
1.3.10.2. poor storage conditions;
1.3.10.3. poor quality product;
1.3.10.4. counterfeit product;
1.3.10.5. interactions.

1.4. Selection of drugs to monitor

1.4.1. It is intended to monitor artemisinin combination therapies (ACTs). A number of these have either already come on to the market or are expected to do so in the near future.

1.4.2. It may be possible to monitor two or more antimalarials under the same conditions and make observations on comparative safety.

1.4.3. Antimalarials other than ACTs can also be monitored if desired for comparison.

1.5. Basic processes

1.5.1. Establishing a cohort of patients for each drug and/or drug combination.

1.5.2. Recording adverse events experienced by patients in the cohort(s) for a defined period.

1.6. Programme duration

1.6.1. CEM is done for a limited length of time. The length depends on the time it takes to achieve the cohort size that is necessary and this will depend on the incidence of malaria in the population being studied. The target sample size is usually around 10 000 patients.

1.6.2. If there is particular interest in certain subgroups e.g. pregnant women or children or those who experience an event of concern, then monitoring may need to continue for a longer period to get sufficient numbers to evaluate these subgroups at a satisfactory level of statistical significance.

1.6.3. A practical approach is to review the data monthly. Trends will be observed that may indicate the need for an extension of monitoring.

2. Epidemiology

The key epidemiological features of CEM studies are that they are:

2.1. Observational

This means that the studies are "*non-interventional*" and are undertaken in real-life situations. Patients are not selected according to any criteria: all patients who are treated for malaria with the medicine being monitored are included. This includes patients of all ages, those with other diseases and those on other medicines. Treatment is given according to the usual local guidelines.

2.2. Prospective

This means that the monitoring is planned before the patients are treated and the patients are studied and followed up from the time they begin their treatment.

2.3. Inceptional

This has a similar meaning to prospective: that every patient is studied from the time of commencement of their treatment.

2.4. Dynamic

This means that new patients are added as the study continues until such time as there are sufficient numbers in the cohort.

2.5. Longitudinal

This means that the patients are studied over a period of time. For antimalarials used for acute treatment this is a matter of only a few days although monitoring may continue longer if looking for delayed effects.

2.6. Descriptive

In terms of a CEM malaria study, this means that the events are identified and described, their frequency is measured and their distribution in different subgroups of the cohort is recorded.

3. First step – Implementation

The implementation step has to be done well if a CEM study is to succeed. It is necessary to do the following:

3.1. Appoint a full-time CEM coordinator.

3.2. Aim at having an initial pilot study.

3.3. Select appropriate sentinel sites, with trained teams and adequate resources to perform CEM.

3.4. Using the most appropriate means, all stakeholders must be fully informed of:

3.4.1. The reasons for monitoring (see 3.5).

3.4.2. The methodology as it involves them.

3.4.3. The value of safety monitoring and the advantages of CEM.

3.4.4. The contribution it will make to the health of the population (improving benefit and reducing risk).

3.4.5. The potential for increasing the effectiveness of public health programmes.

3.4.6. The potential for reducing health costs for the community and government.

3.4.7. The contribution CEM studies in any particular country can make to the knowledge of antimalarials and their safety internationally.

3.5. The reasons for monitoring

The following objectives need to be emphasized as the motivation for providing the data requested. They are similar to the objectives in D.1.3, but have a promotional emphasis rather than a descriptive one.

3.5.1. The earliest possible recognition of new adverse reactions, including interactions.

3.5.2. To measure risk (incidence), including comparative risk of different antimalarials.

3.5.3. To identify risk factors for the important reactions so that they can be avoided in the therapeutic management of malaria and the risk of harm minimized.

3.5.4. To assess safety in pregnancy and lactation.

3.5.5. To provide evidence for:

3.5.5.1. effective risk management;

3.5.5.2. safer use of antimalarials;

3.5.5.3. benefit/harm assessment of different products;

3.5.5.4. evidence-based regulatory action.

3.5.6. To provide cohorts for the future study of new safety concerns.

3.6. Approaches – these need to be adapted for the target audience.

3.6.1. Personal meetings with people of influence in government and the ministry of health, academic institutions, hospitals, public health programmes, WHO offices, professional associations, the pharmaceutical industry, the privacy commissioner, the community and the media.

3.6.2. Presentations at meetings to professional groups e.g. hospital doctors, nurses and pharmacists. This is best achieved at one of their regular meetings.

3.6.3. Produce and distribute leaflets for health professionals and patients.

3.6.4. Produce posters for patients and the community and distribute them to hospitals and clinics.

3.6.5. Cultivate good relationships with key media journalists on newspapers, magazines, radio and television and discuss your work as a newsworthy activity.

3.6.6. Encourage a feeling of collegiality and collaboration in the interests of the health of the community, rather than taking an authoritarian approach.

3.6.7. Develop the detailed application of CEM methodology in consultation with the health workers in the hospitals and clinics.

4. Second step – establishing the cohort(s)

4.1. Numbers of patients

4.1.1. Total numbers

4.1.1.1. See section D.1.6.

4.1.1.2. In general, the aim is to have 10 000 patients in the cohort. This gives a 95% chance of identifying a specific event with an incidence of 1:3000 (uncommon or rare). Normally several events are needed to alert to a signal, or help evaluate a problem.

4.1.1.3. A cohort of 3000 patients gives a 95% chance of identifying a single event with an incidence of 1:1000.

4.1.1.4. If a comparator study is being undertaken, greater numbers will be needed if the background incidence in the community is high (as with diarrhoea) and it may be desirable to detect statistically significant differences between the comparators.

4.1.1.5. Concomitant medicines: larger numbers might be needed to detect differences in patients on specific medicines (e.g. antiretrovirals) compared with the other patients.

4.1.1.6. Other health problems e.g. malnutrition: larger numbers might be needed to detect differences in these patients.

4.1.1.7. Table 1 is useful for deciding on numbers, or estimating the statistical probability of a result with a particular number of patients.

Table 1. **Relationship between sample size and probability of observing an adverse event (AE)**

Per cent probability of observing at least one AE in the sample by AE expected incidence

Sample size	Expected AE incidence: 1 event out of ... patients						
	100	**200**	**500**	**1 000**	**2 000**	**5 000**	**10 000**
200	86.47	63.21	32.97	18.13	9.52	3.92	1.98
300	95.02	77.69	45.12	25.92	13.93	5.82	2.96
500	99.33	91.79	63.21	39.35	22.12	9.52	4.88
700	99.91	96.98	75.34	50.34	29.53	13.06	6.76
1 000	100.00	99.33	86.47	63.21	39.35	18.13	9.52
1 500	100.00	99.94	95.02	77.69	52.76	25.92	13.93
2 000	100.00	100.00	98.17	86.47	63.21	32.97	18.13
3 000	100.00	100.00	99.75	95.02	77.69	45.12	25.92
5 000	100.00	100.00	100.00	99.33	91.79	63.21	39.35
7 000	100.00	100.00	100.00	99.91	96.98	75.34	50.34
10 000	100.00	100.00	100.00	100.00	99.33	86.47	63.21
12 000	100.00	100.00	100.00	100.00	99.75	90.93	69.88
15 000	100.00	100.00	100.00	100.00	99.94	95.02	77.69

As can be seen, a sample size of 3000 patients gives a 95% probability of identifying a particular adverse event, but mostly, for a meaningful assessment, at least three events need to be identified. Hence, the higher objective of obtaining a sample of 10 000 patients. However, the identification of one serious event can be clinically significant.

In relation to the comparison of two medicines, a further two tables and a graph are presented in Annex XV as a guide to the cohort numbers required to reach sufficient statistical power to identify significant differences in the incidence of particular events. The minimum acceptable statistical power is usually 80%.

- Table 1 shows the sample sizes required to identify statistically significant differences when the incidence is 0.1% (1:1000) in one of the comparators.
- Table 2 shows the power that can be achieved with different cohort sizes when the incidence of the event of interest in one of the comparators is 1%.

- The graph demonstrates the power that can be achieved at different levels of difference (RR) for comparison of an event in two medicines with cohort sizes of 1500.

The above demonstrate that the lower the incidence of an event, the larger the cohort needed to identify statistically significant differences when other factors affecting the sample size are kept unchanged.

The tables can be used in two ways:

- To estimate the cohort sizes needed to achieve satisfactory power at particular rates of an event and what level of difference (Relative Risk) is necessary;
- To see what cohorts of a particular size can achieve to demonstrate differences at sufficient power and at what level of difference (RR) between two medicines.

4.1. Selection of patients

4.1.1. Logistics

4.1.1.1. Decisions will need to be made as to where the patients will be recruited and the monitoring to be performed:

• The patients might be recruited from all health facilities involved in the malaria programme.

• Patients might be recruited from selected health facilities that are representative of the whole country, designated as "sentinel monitoring sites".

4.1.1. Inceptional

Patients must be monitored from the *inception* of treatment (see section D.2.3). Patients not seen at the beginning of treatment should be excluded from the study.

4.1.2. Subgroups of interest

4.1.2.1. Children: In order to determine any risk factors specific to children, the whole population of users will still need to be monitored to enable comparison of children with the adults in the cohort, and to detect risk factors specific to children.

4.1.2.2. HIV/AIDS: In order to determine any risk factors specific to patients with HIV/AIDS, the whole population of users will still need to be monitored to enable comparison with the cohort members who do not have HIV/AIDS.

4.1.2.3. Pregnancy: If the only interest in monitoring was in outcomes with pregnancy, then patient selection could be restricted to women of child-bearing age.

4.2. Patient identification

4.2.1. See section C.6.1.1.

4.2.2. It is vital that patients can be identified accurately. Inaccurate identification will result in:

4.2.2.1. duplicate entries in the database leading to inflated numbers in the cohort and inaccurate statistics;

4.2.2.2. difficulties in follow-up.

4.3. Other patient data

4.3.1. Age at the time of treatment. (date of birth to help identification).

4.3.2. Sex.

4.3.3. Weight and height.

4.4. Background data

4.4.1. History of significant illness (e.g. liver disease, kidney disease).

4.4.2. Other diseases present at the time of treatment (e.g. HIV/AIDS, tuberculosis, anaemia).

4.5. Controls or comparators

4.5.1. *Proper control cohorts* would require preselected matches for the patients in a study done under the same conditions at the same time as the study cohort. This would create an artificial situation and it would no longer be an observational (non-interventional) study.

4.5.2. Comparator cohorts. A CEM study of two (or more) antimalarials, given to patients on a random basis for acute malaria over the same study period in the same population, would provide a useful comparison of the medicines involved. Because the patients in the different cohorts are not strict controls, comparisons would have to be made with caution due to the likely presence of confounders.

4.5.3. Pretreatment control period. Adverse events can be recorded for a period before antimalarial treatment is started and for the same period after treatment, for each patient. The events recorded before treatment would serve as an accurate control for the events occurring after treatment. This would be the most satisfactory method of controlling for background noise. The aim of monitoring, therefore, is to record any adverse events occurring during the week following treatment as well as events occurring in the week before treatment, i.e. in the pretreatment control period.

5. Third step – acquiring the data

The medicines

5.1. Details of administration of antimalarial medicine

5.1.1. The following should be recorded:

5.1.1.1. brand name, e.g. Coartem;

5.1.1.2. dose and schedule of administration;

5.1.1.3. date of commencement of treatment;

5.1.1.4. date of completion of course of therapy or date of withdrawal;

5.1.1.5. record of incomplete adherence;

5.1.1.6. record reason(s) for incomplete adherence.

5.2. Concomitant medicines

5.2.1. All medicines taken during the 2 weeks prior to treatment and at any time from day 0 of treatment until the follow-up appointment should be recorded (first day of treatment is day 0).

5.2.2. Record the following information on concomitant medicines:

5.2.2.1. name: brand (preferred) or generic;

5.2.2.2. any traditional medicine(s) ("yes" or "no");

5.2.2.3. indication for use;

5.2.2.4. dose and frequency of administration;

5.2.2.5. date started;

5.2.2.6. date stopped (record "continues" if not stopped).

The events

5.3. Principles of event reporting

5.3.1. All adverse events are requested to be reported and not just suspected adverse reactions. Clinicians should be asked to make no judgement on causality.

5.3.2. "Adverse events" are requested to be reported because there are always unexpected or unrecognized adverse reactions. If only suspected reactions are reported, then those which are unexpected and unrecognized are likely to be missed.

5.3.3. All clinical events experienced by each patient should be recorded on the questionnaire provided. This includes unexpected improvement of concomitant disease (favourable event) as well as adverse events.

5.3.4. Pretreatment: Each patient who attends a health care facility with an attack of malaria should be asked if any health events have occurred in the previous 7 days and these should be recorded as having occurred during the control period. These should include diseases such as otitis media, tonsillitis, measles and abscess.

5.3.5. Post-treatment: At the follow-up visit any *new* events or worsening of pre-existing conditions that have occurred since treatment began should be recorded.

5.4. Reporting requirements

Health professionals should be asked to record the following types of events:

5.4.1. All *new* events even if minor.

5.4.2. Change in a pre-existing condition.

5.4.3. Abnormal changes in laboratory tests.

5.4.4. Persistent positive tests for malaria.

5.4.5. Admission to hospital with date and cause.

5.4.6. Pregnancy of any duration.

5.4.7. Accidents.

5.4.8. All deaths with date and cause.

5.4.9. Possible interactions.

5.4.9.1. Include pharmaceutical or traditional medicines.

5.4.9.2. Remember oral contraceptives and alcohol.

5.4.9.3. Be aware of the possibility of food–drug interactions.

5.5. Recording event details

A brief description of each event is usually all that is necessary. These event descriptions will be reviewed later by pharmacovigilance staff and standard adverse event terminology will be applied by them. The clinician does not need to know the standard event terminology.

5.6. Reporting forms (questionnaires)

5.6.1. The CEM questionnaires have two sides (see Annex 1)

5.6.1.1. Side A is the Pretreatment questionnaire. This information is used to record patient details, treatment and the events during the pretreatment control period.

5.6.1.2. Side B is the post-treatment (or follow-up) questionnaire. This provides the follow-up informa-

tion on events and outcomes of treatment since treatment began.

5.6.2. It is important to make the recording of data as easy as possible. Remember that this is an additional task that you are asking busy health professionals to undertake while working in a busy clinic.

5.6.3. The patient details should be recorded by an assistant before the patient is seen by the clinical worker.

5.6.4. The questionnaire may need to be adapted for local use.

5.6.5. Consideration should be given to printing the questionnaires on duplicate self-copying (NCR) paper.

5.6.5.1. There would need to be a "pad A" for questionnaire A and "pad B" for questionnaire B.

5.6.5.2. It would be an advantage to have them colour-coded.

5.6.5.3. When completed, the top copy of each form should be sent to the Pharmacovigilance Centre and the duplicate copy retained in the health facility with the patient's record, where possible, or in another convenient location.

5.6.5.4. Questionnaire A would then be sent to the Pharmacovigilance Centre, according to local procedures, without waiting for questionnaire B to be completed.

5.6.5.5. This policy should result in a reduced likelihood that forms will be lost; copies of the questionnaires would be retained in the health facility for reference; questionnaire A would reach the Pharmacovigilance Centre earlier and the data manager for the CEM programme would have the opportunity to identify patients who failed to return for follow-up in addition to the follow-up check at the health facility.

5.7. Who should report?

5.7.1. Health workers with clinical responsibility should record the events.

5.7.2. It is desirable that the health worker who treated the patient at the first visit should also see the patient at follow-up.

5.8. Follow-up

5.8.1. At the time of treatment and enrolment in the study, each patient should be given a follow-up appointment for monitoring purposes and asked to return 7 days later in order to record any adverse events. A shorter period of follow-up could lead to important developing adverse events, e.g. hepatic reactions being missed. Normal practice for the health facility should be continued in regard to clinical follow-up, which is often after 3–5 days.

5.8.2. Assistance to support compliance with follow-up should be considered, e.g. payment of travel costs or supply of treated mosquito nets.

5.8.3. When the patient returns to the health facility, the same clinician who made the pre-treatment assessment should, in principle, also be responsible for making the post-treatment evaluation.

5.8.4. Defaulters should be actively traced at home/village level by visits of support staff who will interview the patient or carer and refer back all patients presenting with "new events, even if minor" or "deterioration in a pre-existing condition". A special form for patient tracking should be drawn up, with the following information:

5.8.4.1. patient identification;

5.8.4.2. date of home/follow-up visit;

5.8.4.3. name of health worker;

5.8.4.4. outcome of visit, indicating:

- *no new event;*
- *improvement of clinical condition;*
- *the presence of new adverse events and subsequent referral to the treatment centre for clinical assessment;*
- *reasons for referral.*

5.8.5. The timing of follow-up of defaulters should be no later than 7 days after the missed follow-up appointment.

5.8.6. Events that become obvious after the 7-day follow-up period, and which appear to be reactions to the ACT, should be reported on a spontaneous reporting form.

5.8.6.1. To facilitate this, spontaneous reporting forms should be stamped 'CEM' and placed, where possible, with the patient's record, or otherwise be readily available in the health facility.

5.8.6.2. Completed and stamped CEM forms should be sent to the CEM programme coordinator in the Pharmacovigilance Centre, so that the events data can be added to the patient's details in the CEM database.

5.9. Reasons for non-adherence

It is important to record any of the following, or other reasons, for non-adherence to the treatment schedule.

5.9.1. Persistent vomiting.

5.9.2. Other adverse events.

5.9.3. Patient felt better quickly.

5.9.4. Patient felt worse (possible inadequate response).

5.9.5. Patient wished to keep some of the tablets.

5.10. How and where to send the completed questionnaires

5.10.1. The completed questionnaires need to be sent to the National Pharmacovigilance Centre where the events will be assessed and the information entered into a database.

5.10.2. The method of sending the questionnaires needs to be planned with each health facility, from hospitals to rural clinics.

5.10.2.1. It may be desirable for rural clinics to send their reports to district hospitals and for district hospitals to send them to referral hospitals which will send them to the Pharmacovigilance Centre. However, some other method may suit local circumstances better. An appropriate chain of communica-

tion needs to be established and everyone involved should be well informed about it.

5.10.2.2. The questionnaires should be stored securely so that they cannot be accessed by unauthorized people.

5.10.2.3. An appropriate frequency for sending the reports needs to be established, e.g. weekly, and the role of checking on the transfer of the reports along the chain needs to be assigned to a suitable person.

5.11. Record linkage

Record linkage is another method of active surveillance that may be used to supplement or check information received on the CEM questionnaires.

5.11.1. This is a method of searching different health databases electronically using unique patient identifiers.

5.11.2. The unique patient identifiers (or national health numbers) must be in use nationally to enable national registers of deaths or diseases to be searched. The identifying health number must be recorded with the patient details in the cohort database.

5.11.3. Examples of databases that may be available for searching using the health identifiers are:

5.11.3.1. register of deaths;

5.11.3.2. register of congenital abnormalities;

5.11.3.3. cancer registers;

5.11.3.4. other specialist registers, e.g. myocardial infarction.

5.11.4. In the absence of national numbers, other identifying numbers (e.g. hospital numbers) if available, can be recorded in the patient cohort data. It would then be possible to use these numbers to search registers maintained by the hospital (e.g. a teaching hospital) or another facility that has health (or disease) registers.

6. Database for CEM

6.1. Choice of database

6.1.1. There is no readily available database for immediate use for CEM. The IMMP and PEM in the UK have developed their own databases, but these might not be suitable for monitoring antimalarials.

6.1.2. Microsoft Access could be used, but is difficult to manage and not wholly satisfactory.

6.1.3. Purpose-built databases can be programmed using SAS (the commercially available Statistical Analysis System). This requires a person with expertise in this software.

6.1.4. A relational database is desirable that can link separate smaller databases for analysis as required. A single database with all the data would be too big to manage.

6.1.5. An adaptation of VigiFlow for CEM would be ideal. The UMC is currently developing this tool.

6.2. Data elements/fields

6.2.1. It is desirable to have separate databases for:

6.2.1.1. the cohorts with all patient data;

6.2.1.2. the medicines with all details of use;

6.2.1.3. the events with dates and outcomes;

6.2.1.4. the reporters (treatment providers) with contact details.

6.2.2. Fields required in the database need to allow for entry of all the data elements included on the questionnaires.

6.2.3. Data elements included are:

6.2.3.1. Patient

- *name;*
- *clinic and/or study numbers and/or national ID health number;*
- *address or contact details;*

- *gender;*
- *date of birth and/or age;*
- *weight and height;*
- *pregnancy status, if applicable.*

6.2.3.2. Medicine(s)

- *WHO Drug Dictionary name and ATC code;*
- *indication for use (ICD-10 code);*
- *dose;*
- *date of commencement;*
- *quantity supplied;*
- *instructions for use;*
- *date of stopping treatment;*
- *date of withdrawal*
- *date of dose reduction;*
- *date of rechallenge ; and*
- *concomitant medicines with details of administration and dates.*

6.2.3.3 Events (see sections D.1.1. and D.5.3.)

- *event term(s);*
- *print code (see section D.9.3.);*
- *date of onset;*
- *effect of dechallenge;*
- *effect of rechallenge;*
- *severity;*
- *seriousness;*
- *outcome;*
- *relationship.*

6.2.3.4 Contact details of treatment provider/reporter

- *name;*
- *status (doctor, nurse, etc);*
- *hospital or clinic name, telephone and fax number.*

7. Maximizing the reporting rate

7.1. In all the planning phases and communications with health professionals, health workers and public health staff, it is important to try to develop a culture of collaboration: working together for the successful management of malaria in the safest possible way for the patients.

7.2. Removing barriers to reporting. The following means of removing barriers need to be considered:

7.2.1. Ensure an adequate supply of readily available questionnaires.

7.2.2. Make sure everyone is adequately briefed on the importance and value of CEM and understands the basic methodology.

7.2.3. Minimize the recording requirements for clinicians. Have assistants do as much recording as possible before the clinician sees the patient.

7.2.4. Don't ask for information that is not absolutely necessary.

7.2.5. Don't ask for information that might take a long time to find, e.g. batch numbers, unless it is very important.

7.3. Feedback. Good feedback will encourage compliance by the health professionals and health workers. They will need regular information to be sent to them by the Pharmacovigilance Centre. This information needs to be relevant and helpful to their work. Occasional meetings to discuss the results are valuable.

8. General advice and information

8.1. Don't ask for too much

8.1.1. The more you ask for the less you will get.

8.1.2. Assess the necessity for every data item requested.

8.1.3. Increased data increases the workload and the cost.

8.1.4. Some information is best requested by follow-up when the necessity for it can be explained and interest created by the problem being explored.

8.2. Non-serious events

It is important to include these because:

8.2.1. They might indicate a serious problem.

8.2.2. They might affect adherence, e.g. nausea.

8.2.3. If common, they might be more important to public health than rare, but serious problems.

8.3. Be open-minded

8.3.1. Predictions of safety, if based only on spontaneous reporting, are unreliable.

8.3.2. Unexpected reactions will occur.

8.3.3. Avoid pre-conceived ideas.

8.3.4. All data should be collected and analysed in a totally *objective* manner.

8.4. Privacy

8.4.1. Given basic precautions to maintain confidentiality, patients give greater priority to safety concerns.

8.4.2. Security and confidentiality of data is the essential requirement. Other ethical requirements should not prevent CEM taking place or reduce its functionality, because it is unethical not to pursue those methods that are essential to safety assessment and the protection of patients.

8.4.3. Ethical issues are discussed in section M.2.

9. Fourth step – Clinical review

This involves the following activities in the Pharmacovigilance Centre:

- Assessing the clinical details and determining the appropriate event terms.
- Determining the duration to onset of each event.
- Recording data on dechallenge and rechallenge (if any).
- Determining severity and seriousness.
- Recording the outcome of each event.
- Undertaking a relationship assessment for each event as the first step in establishing causality.

9.1. The event should be specific to be acceptable for recording

For example, sometimes a "stomach upset" is reported, but this description is too vague. It could mean dyspepsia, nausea, vomiting, diarrhoea, or some other specific event.

9.2. Determining the event term

9.2.1. A person with clinical expertise (the CEM Clinical Supervisor) in the Pharmacovigilance Centre should review the details of the events described.

9.2.2. The first decision to be made is which clinical group(s), e.g. alimentary or respiratory, would be the most appropriate in which to record the event(s).

9.2.3. The most appropriate term should then be selected from the particular system organ class (SOC) in the WHO-ART dictionary.

9.2.4. The selected terms should be recorded for later data entry on a coding sheet (see section E.3.4 and Annex 2).

9.3. Building an events dictionary

The need for an *events* dictionary arises because the readily available dictionaries are *reaction* dictionaries related to the spontaneous reporting of suspected adverse reactions rather than of *events*.

9.3.0.1. Event monitoring requires a dictionary of clinical events, many of which will not be reactions.

9.3.0.2. Clinical events need to be recorded in order to identify unexpected reactions.

9.3.0.3. Event monitoring of new medicines in developing countries will produce many new event terms because of:

- *the different medicines being used, e.g. ACTs;*
- *the different diseases being treated (for the purposes of this manual, malaria);*
- *the different pattern of background morbidity e.g. parasitic diseases, a high incidence of HIV/AIDS and malnutrition;*
- *different concomitant medicines;*
- *different ethnicity, diet and living conditions.*

9.3.1. The purposes of building an *events* dictionary are as follows:

9.3.1.1. to develop a standardized terminology that can be used for international comparisons of results;

9.3.1.2. as a tool for collating the events in clinically meaningful groupings;

9.3.1.3. to help create a clinical collation of events that enables a visualization of the pattern of morbidity in the cohort and community;

9.3.1.4. to present a clinical collation of events that provides a key to rapid signal identification.

9.3.2. Essential requirements of an events dictionary are:

9.3.2.1. that it has a structure that will present the event terms in clinically related groupings;

9.3.2.2. that it is rapidly adaptable to meet the day-to-day needs of the event monitoring programmes.

9.3.3. Creating a clinical order

9.3.3.1. The first step is to list the Clinical Categories.

9.3.3.2. The Clinical Categories are similar to the System Organ Classes (SOCs) in the WHO-ART dictionary with some adaptation to allow for the specific needs of CEM, e.g. a pregnancy register. (see Annex 3).

9.3.3.3. Where possible, individual terms should be selected from WHO-ART.

9.3.3.4. Because WHO-ART is a reaction dictionary and not an event dictionary, an appropriate event term may not be available and will need to be selected from some other source. Recognized terms that have dictionary definitions are most likely to be found in a medical textbook. It is important to choose terms that have precise meanings. A good source that includes terms from medical specialties is The Merck Manual of General Medicine and Specialties. The IMMP events dictionary may be available as a reference and suitable terms might be found in ICD-10 or MedDRA.

9.3.3.5. The Council for International Organizations of Medical Sciences (CIOMS) has published a very useful reference for defined reaction terms (see references in Annex 12).

9.3.3.6. Each term that is added to the dictionary should be given a "print code". These codes create a structure that allows the events to be sorted in the required clinical order. This will include subgroups that do the best clinical sort of the events data.

9.3.3.7. The event dictionary print codes are not to be entered instead of the event name, because the codes may change to accommodate the addition of new terms. They are recorded to enable the events to be sorted in a clinically meaningful way. Therefore, the event names need to be entered as well as the codes.

9.3.3.8. An ideal solution for a CEM events dictionary would be to have it available for access in the CEM adaptation of VigiFlow.

9.3.3.9. For a listing of the Clinical Categories and a sample page of the IMMP events dictionary see Annexes 3 and 4.

9.3.3.10. New terms may be added by the administrators of individual programmes, but when the reports with new terms are forwarded to the UMC, these new terms will be flagged for consideration by a central standardizing committee, which will give feed-back on the terms approved.

9.4. Seriousness

9.4.1. This is defined in section C.2 and C.6.2.2 and each event should be routinely recorded as either serious or not serious.

9.4.2. If serious, then the reason for this choice of description should be given. The coding sheet allows for a code to be entered, e.g. "H" for hospitalized or prolonged hospitalization.

9.5. Severity

9.5.1. Severity does not have the same meaning as seriousness. A patient can experience a severe event that is not serious e.g. pruritus.

9.5.2. Severity is a subjective assessment made by the patient and/or the clinician. Although subjective, it is nevertheless useful in identifying reactions that may affect adherence.

9.5.3. It can be recorded on the coding sheet as "1" for severe or "2" for not severe.

9.6. Outcome

9.6.1. The types of outcome to be recorded are listed on the coding sheet (with codes for entry), and are:

- recovered without sequelae;
- recovered with sequelae;
- not yet recovered;
- died due to adverse reaction;
- died – medicine may be contributory;
- died – unrelated to medicine;
- died – cause unknown.

9.6.2. Normally recording the outcome is a matter of recording the outcome entered on the questionnaire, but at times clinical judgement is required, e.g. when recording deaths.

9.7. Relationship: This is discussed in section G.

E. Data processing

1. Data entry

1.1. Requirements

1.1.1. Data must be accurate.

1.1.2. Data processors must be trained and supervised until they are confident of their level of skill.

1.1.3. Data processors need to be given good tools (a good computer and suitable office furniture). It is an exacting job.

1.1.4. Share the vision and share the results with the data processors. Help them to see that they are a vital part of the team.

1.2. Standard formats

The use of standard formats is a means of reducing error.

1.2.1. Methods

1.2.1.1. Use input masks so that anything other than predetermined terms will be rejected.

1.2.1.2. Use field controls so that certain values can only be entered in a selected way.

1.2.1.3. Use drop-down lists for standard choices.

1.2.2. Examples

1.2.2.1. Date format: dd/mm/yy.

1.2.2.2. Numbers: restrict number of digits to what is appropriate for values entered into particular fields, e.g. age – restrict to 2 digits.

1.2.2.3. Use Anatomic Therapeutic Classification (ATC) codes for medicines and ICD-10 codes for diseases.

1.2.2.4. Drop-down lists: use M or F for sex; doses – mg, ml, etc; names of hospitals and clinics.

2. Quality control

2.1. Control at entry

2.1.1. Use field controls and standard formats as in E.1.2.

2.1.2. The use of codes, e.g. ICD-10 or ATC codes results in fewer errors than does typing in names.

2.2. Systematic checks

2.2.1. Print lists of data regularly e.g. every morning or every week (depending on the volume of data) and do a manual check of the different fields. Examples of what to look for include:

2.2.1.1. dates that are improbable;

2.2.1.2. male sex with female name;

2.2.1.3. similar names (e.g. Joe and Joseph) with the same date of birth who could be the same patient.

2.2.2. Sort the data by important fields in turn and check each printout.

2.2.3. Apparent inaccuracies need to be checked against the original data and corrected where necessary.

2.2.4. The computer counts slight differences separately and will inflate the numbers if there are duplications due to inaccuracies.

3. Coding of medicines and diseases

3.1. Use the ATC classification for medicines.

3.2. Use the ICD-10 for diseases that are recorded as indications for treatment or diseases recorded in the medical history. (The ICD is also a useful source of acceptable event names).

3.3. These codes are accessible in VigiFlow and will be available in the adaptation for CEM.

3.4. Standardized recording of event details

3.4.1. A *coding sheet* is a useful tool for reviewing the clinical details in a report. An example is provided in Annex 2.

3.4.2. Use of a coding sheet by reviewers ensures a systematic and standard approach to reviewing the events described on the questionnaires.

3.4.3. The coding sheet should be completed before data entry. This facilitates data entry, reduces error and reduces the time online.

3.4.4. When the CEM adaptation of Vigiflow is in use, a coding sheet will no longer be necessary.

3.5. Collating and summarizing the events

3.5.1. This should be done at regular intervals during CEM – at least monthly.

3.5.2. The events are sorted by the event print codes in the dictionary.

3.5.3. When a printout is made, the events listing will reveal the clinical pattern of the events occurring with the drug being studied in the local environment.

3.5.4. This events collation should incorporate the following fields:

3.5.4.1. event

3.5.4.2. sex

3.5.4.3. age

3.5.4.4. dose

3.5.4.5. duration to onset in days, hours or minutes

3.5.4.6. relationship, coded as follows: 1 (certain), 2 (probable), 3 (possible), 4 (unlikely), 5 (unclassified), 6 (unclassifiable)

3.5.4.7. report number

3.5.4.8. death

3.5.4.9. withdrawal.

3.5.5. The collation will be the main means of identifying signals simply by observing the clinical patterns.

3.5.6. A sample page of collated events can be seen in Annex 5.

3.5.7. Constructing event/risk profiles:

3.5.7.1. This is done by graphically representing the rates of events in each Clinical Category, but can also be performed on groups of related events within a Category.

3.5.7.2. It is particularly useful for comparing two or more medicines.

3.5.7.3. A sample page of comparative event profiles can be seen in Annex 6.

3.5.7.4. To develop a risk profile, only those events coded as having a relationship of 1, 2 or 3 should be included. This results in a profile of those events with a plausible relationship and illustrates the actual risk pattern better than an events profile which includes all events, including those with an "unlikely" relationship.

F. Special types of event

1. Serious events

1.1. These are defined in sections C.2 and C.6.2.2. See also D.9.4.

1.2. Details of serious events should be sent immediately to the Pharmacovigilance Centre where they will be fully assessed and appropriate action taken.

1.3. A process needs to be defined for each health facility to follow so that there is no delay. national drug regulatory authorities often have in place standard operating procedures and clear timelines for transmission of case-report forms in case of serious adverse events. Regulatory requirements for reporting should be integrated into the procedures for CEM.

2. Pregnancies

2.1. Background

2.1.1. "Pregnant women with symptomatic acute malaria are a high risk group. Malaria in pregnancy is associated with low birth weight, increased anaemia, and in low transmission areas, an increased risk of severe malaria…". (*WHO Guidelines for the treatment of malaria.* 2006: p 32–34).

2.1.2. Artemisinin derivatives should be used to treat uncomplicated falciparum malaria in the second and third trimesters, but should not be used in the first trimester until more information becomes available.

2.1.3. A very important aspect of CEM of ACTs is obtaining more information on safety in pregnancy, particularly following inadvertent exposure during the first trimester.

2.1.4. The success of obtaining outcomes of exposure during pregnancy depends on the adequacy of follow-up.

2.1.5. Strenuous efforts need to be made to identify those women who were inadvertently exposed to ACTs during the first trimester.

2.2. Follow-up

2.2.1. Three follow-up questionnaires have been designed to facilitate the gathering of outcome information following exposure to ACTs during pregnancy.

2.2.1.1. Pregnancy Enquiry Questionnaire Annex 7A.

2.2.1.2. Pregnancy Progress Questionnaire Annex 7B.

2.2.1.3. Pregnancy Outcome Questionnaire Annex 7C.

2.2.2. All women who are known to be pregnant at the time of receiving an ACT should be followed up to find out the outcome of the pregnancy and the health status of the infant.

2.2.2.1. A standard operating procedure needs to be developed for each health facility to ensure that every woman known to be pregnant is followed up by a health worker using the Pregnancy Progress Questionnaire and the Pregnancy Outcome Questionnaire.

2.2.2.2. Coordination and collaboration should be developed with antenatal clinics and birthing units.

2.2.3. An attempt should be made to identify all women who were subject to inadvertent exposure to ACT during the first trimester:

2.2.3.1. Each woman of child-bearing age (14–50 years) in the cohort of patients treated with ACTs, should be followed up 4–5 months after treatment in order to enquire about the likelihood of having been pregnant at the time of treatment.

2.2.3.2. This may be done by routine domiciliary visits, or by giving women an appointment to return in 4 months and then visiting only the defaulters. This latter option might reduce the number of home visits required.

2.2.3.3. The Pregnancy Enquiry Questionnaire (Annex 7A) should be completed at this patient contact.

2.2.3.4. The possibility of performing pregnancy tests at the routine follow-up at 7 days post-treat-

ment should be considered. This would give more reliable results and is likely to be more cost-effective than making home visits at 4–5 months after treatment, but would require ethical approval.

2.2.3.5. A standard operating procedure needs to be developed for each health facility to ensure that every woman identified as pregnant is followed up by a health worker using the Pregnancy Progress Questionnaire and the Pregnancy Outcome Questionnaire.

2.2.4. At delivery and/or a postnatal visit, the Pregnancy Outcome Questionnaire should be completed. The recommended questionnaire is reproduced in Annex 7C.

2.2.4.1. A standard operating procedure needs to be developed for each health facility to ensure that the Pregnancy Outcome Questionnaire is completed for every woman in the cohort who has given birth and that it is returned to the Pharmacovigilance Centre.

2.2.4.2. Coordination and collaboration should be developed with the birthing units.

2.3. Pregnancy Register

2.3.1. If a woman is found to be pregnant at the 7 day follow-up visit, this should be recorded as an event on the *Post-treatment Questionnaire B* and will then be entered into the database when the questionnaire is returned to the Pharmacovigilance Centre.

2.3.2. If pregnancy is confirmed later, as in section 2.2.3, the information will be entered into the database from the pregnancy questionnaires.

2.3.3. The most convenient way of compiling a pregnancy register is to put details of all pregnancies into the special Clinical Category, *"Pregnancy exposure"* in the events database. This category should be reviewed with the regular general collation of events and as required.

2.3.4. The fields that should be incorporated in the pregnancy register are:

2.3.4.1. duration of pregnancy on date of exposure;

2.3.4.2. outcome of pregnancy;

2.3.4.3. duration of pregnancy at birth;

2.3.4.4. outcome for fetus or newborn;

2.3.4.5. age of mother;

2.3.4.6. doses of antimalarial medicine.

2.3.4.7. other medicines taken, including traditional medicines. These data should be sought only if there is an abnormal outcome of pregnancy. It is often difficult to obtain an accurate record because of difficulty of recall, but the details from Questionnaire A and subsequent follow-up pregnancy questionnaires should be available. Records of attendances at the health facility and at antenatal clinics should also be helpful.

2.3.4.8. Report number.

2.3.5. Any congenital abnormalities should be reported immediately to the Pharmacovigilance Centre for further investigation.

2.3.6. The CEM coordinator in the Pharmacovigilance Centre should review the register regularly and ensure that all follow-up procedures have been undertaken, or attempted. A standard operating procedure should be developed for this.

2.4. Lactation exposure

2.4.1. Questions about exposure of the infant during lactation in a woman who has taken antimalarial treatment are included in the pregnancy questionnaire.

2.4.2. At the follow-up appointment 7-days post-treatment, breastfeeding women need to be asked about any events they have observed in their infant.

2.4.3. The outcome for every infant exposed during lactation should be recorded. If there have been no events, it is important to record, "*no effect*" as the outcome.

2.4.4. Details of exposure during lactation should be treated as a special Clinical Category called "*Lactation exposure*" in order to establish a register with outcomes.

2.5. Verification of drug-effect

If congenital abnormalities are noted in any infant, then this finding should be followed up in an attempt to establish causality. This is a specialist activity that should be initiated by the Pharmacovigilance Centre in consultation with its Expert Safety Review Panel (Advisory Committee).[1]

3. Deaths

3.1. All deaths should be followed up to assess the cause, even if it seems most unlikely that death was related to the medicine.

3.2. Deaths should be listed in a special Clinical Category to compile a register for regular review with each collation of events. This facilitates assessment. A sample listing of deaths is included in Annex 8.

3.3. With CEM, death rates can be calculated. This has particular advantages:

3.3.1. Importantly, death rates can be used to measure changes in outcomes.

3.3.2. Death rates can be compared between comparators. Differences may demonstrate greater effectiveness or greater safety, although the numbers in an antimalarial programme are likely to be too small to make a statistically significant assessment..

4. Lack of efficacy

4.1. Event terms

4.1.1. Lack of efficacy should always be recorded. The following WHO-ART terms should be used as appropriate.

4.1.1.1. "medicine ineffective";

4.1.1.2. "therapeutic response decreased".

1 The Expert Safety Review Panel (or Advisory Committee) is a committee of experts that considers important safety issues and gives advice to the Pharmacovigilance Centre and regulatory authority. The committee's composition and role is described in *The safety of medicines in public health programmes: pharmacovigilance an essential tool.* World Health Organization 2006: p. 38.

4.2. Reasons for lack of efficacy

4.2.1. These are important events to record. Possible reasons for lack of effect are as follows:

4.2.1.1. did not retain the medication because of vomiting or severe diarrhoea;

4.2.1.2. lack of adherence to treatment schedule;

4.2.1.3. inadequate dose;

4.2.1.4. poor quality medication;

4.2.1.5. counterfeit medication;

4.2.1.6. incorrect diagnosis;

4.2.1.7. interactions reducing blood levels;

4.2.1.8. drug resistance.

4.3. Recrudescence of malaria

4.3.1. Recrudescence refers to a recurrence of malaria parasitaemia earlier than would be expected after proper treatment. It is defined as the recurrence of asexual parasitaemia after treatment of the infection with the same infection that caused the original illness. This results from incomplete clearance of the parasitaemia by treatment..

4.3.2. "*Recrudescence*" should be recorded as an event if reappearance of parasitaemia occurs within 14 days after the start of full treatment.

4.3.3. Recrudescence of malaria should be recorded as it may represent a decreased therapeutic response due to developing resistance or any of the above.

5. Delayed reactions

5.1. Delayed reactions to ACTs are unlikely to be seen because of the short treatment period and the short period of follow-up.

5.2. The recommended follow-up for event monitoring is one week after commencement of treatment. However it is possible that some important adverse reactions may not become apparent until after this time, e.g. hepatic reactions.

5.3. If delayed reactions are observed after the follow-up appointment, they should be reported on a spontaneous reporting card as described in section D.5.8.6. These later events should be included in the CEM events database together with events reported earlier on the questionnaires.

6. Concomitant morbid conditions

6.1. Patients may be more susceptible to adverse reactions if they also have other health problems, either because of the concomitant condition or from the interaction of malaria medicines with those being used to treat the other illness. The following are examples of concomitant illnesses that may result in such problems:

6.1.1. HIV/AIDS

6.1.2. tuberculosis

6.1.3. malnutrition

6.1.4. anaemia.

6.2. Concomitant conditions should therefore always be recorded and they can then be tested statistically as risk factors.

G. Relationship/Causality assessment

1. Background

1.1. Two basic questions

These questions need to be addressed separately:

1.1.1. Is there a convincing relationship between the drug and the event?

1.1.2. Did the drug actually cause the event?

1.2. Objective and subjective assessments

1.2.1. The objective phase takes into account actual observations and establishes the *relationship* (see sections G.2 and G.4, below).

1.2.2. The subjective phase which follows is that of making

an attempt to establish a firm opinion about *causality* in those events for which a close relationship has been established. It takes into account the plausibility of the drug being the cause of the event, after having considered the (known) pharmacology, other experience with the medicine or related medicines and inferences made from epidemiological observations and statistical evaluations (see section I).

1.3. General understanding

1.3.1. Establishing causality is a process which begins by examining the relationship between the drug and the event.

1.3.2. The relationship of a single case-report can be established, but it may not be possible to establish a firm opinion on causality until a collection of such reports is assessed or new knowledge is gained.

1.3.3. The ultimate goal of assessment of each event, or a cluster of events being treated as a signal, is an answer to the question: *Did the drug cause the event(s)?* (yes or no?).

1.3.4. Causality for individual reports, even those with a close relationship, can seldom be established beyond doubt and our assessments are based on probability.

1.3.5. A causality assessment should be seen as provisional and subject to change in the light of further information on the case, or new knowledge coming from other sources.

2. Factors to consider when assessing the relationship between drug and event

2.1. Did the event begin before the patient commenced the medicine?

This may seem an obvious consideration, but reports are received in which this has not been taken into account, and a careful check has then revealed that the event preceded the use of the suspect medicine and therefore there was no relationship.

2.2. Is there any other possible cause for the event?

2.2.1. Could the event be due to the illness being treated?

2.2.2. Could it be due to some other co-existent disease?

2.2.3. Could it be due to some other medicine being used concurrently?

2.3. Is the duration to onset of the event plausible?

2.3.1. Is the event likely to have occurred in the time frame in question?

2.3.2. Did it occur too quickly to be related to the particular medicine, taking into account its pharmacological action?

2.3.3. Did the patient take the medicine for a long time without any problems? (Delayed reactions after long-term exposure do occur, but most reactions will occur soon after the patient starts to take the medicine.

2.3.4. The nature of the event should be considered when assessing the significance of the period of exposure, e.g.

2.3.4.1. Some events take a long time to develop (e.g. cancer).

2.3.4.2. Some develop quickly (e.g. nausea and headache).

2.3.4.3. Allergic reactions to first-time exposure to a drug generally take around 10 days to appear. On repeat exposure they may occur immediately.

2.4. Did the event occur after the commencement of some other medicine?

If the event began shortly after commencing another medicine, then two possibilities should be considered:

2.4.1. The new medicine may have caused the event.

2.4.2. There may have been an interaction between the two drugs and the interaction caused the event.

2.5. Did the event occur after the onset of some new illness?

If so, the event may be due to the new illness.

2.6. What is the response to withdrawal of the medicine (dechallenge)?

2.6.1. Did the patient recover?

2.6.2. Did the patient improve?

2.6.3. Was there no change?

2.6.4. Did the patient get worse?

2.6.5. Is the response to dechallenge unknown? If this is the case, then it should always be recorded as unknown.

If more than one medicine has been withdrawn, and if rechallenge is considered appropriate, it should be performed with only one medicine at a time. A positive rechallenge means that:

2.6.6. The patient recovered on initial withdrawal.

2.6.7. The patient developed the same problem again when re-exposed to the same medicine alone, although it may be of a different severity.

2.6.8. The patient recovered when the medicine was withdrawn once again.

2.6.9. It should be noted that it is not always safe to subject the patient to a rechallenge.

2.6.10. If the response to rechallenge is unknown, this should be recorded.

3. Categories of relationship

There are six standard categories of relationship between drug and event. These are the same as the causality categories in the WHO International Drug Monitoring Programme.

3.1. certain (or definite);

3.2. probable;

3.3. possible;

3.4. unlikely;

3.5. unclassified (conditional);

3.6. unassessable (unclassifiable).

4. Requirements for inclusion of an event in a specific category:

4.1. Certain

4.1.1. The event is a specific clinical or laboratory phenomenon.

4.1.2. The time elapsed between the administration of the drug and the occurrence of the event is plausible. (*Requirement*: dates of drug administration and date of onset of the event must be known.)

4.1.3. The event cannot be explained by concomitant disease or any other drug or chemical. (*Requirement*: Details of other medicines taken must be known. The report must also state if there were no other medicines in use. If this is unknown, then doubt exists and the event cannot be included in this category.)

4.1.4. The patient recovered within a plausible length of time following withdrawal of the drug. (*Requirement*: The date of withdrawal of the drug and the time taken for recovery should be known. If these dates are unknown, then doubt exists and the event cannot be included in this category.)

4.1.5. The same event recurred following rechallenge with the same drug alone. (*Requirement*: The report must state the outcome of rechallenge. If this is unknown, then doubt exists and the event cannot be included in this category.)

4.2. Probable

4.2.1. The event is a specific clinical or laboratory phenomenon.

4.2.2. The time elapsed between the administration of the drug and the occurrence of the event is plausible. (The dates of drug administration and date of onset of the event must be known.)

4.2.3. The event cannot be explained by concurrent disease or any other drug or chemical. (Details of other medicines taken must be known. The report must also state if there were no other medicines in use. If this is unknown, then doubt exists and the event cannot be included in this category).

4.2.4. The patient recovered within a plausible length of time following withdrawal of the drug. (The date of drug withdrawal and the time taken for recovery should be known.)

4.2.5. Rechallenge did not occur, or the result is unknown.

4.3. Possible

4.3.1. The time elapsed between the administration of the drug and the occurrence of the event is plausible. (The dates of drug administration and date of onset of the event must be known.)

4.3.2. The outcome of withdrawal of the suspect medicine might not be known, or the medicine might have been continued and the final outcome is not known.

4.3.3. There might be no information on withdrawal of the medicine.

4.3.4. The event could be explained by concomitant disease or use of other drugs or chemicals.

4.3.5. There might be no information on the presence or absence of other medicines.

4.3.6. Deaths cannot be coded as probable because there is no opportunity to see the effect of withdrawal of the drug. If there is a plausible time relationship, a death should be coded as possible.

4.3.7. In addition to deaths, there is a further group of events that do not fit the relationship assessment process and the coding can vary. Consider the following examples:

> *4.3.7.1. Myocardial infarction. Many patients recover from this event as part of the natural history of the disease and, with very few exceptions, recovery is not a response to withdrawal of a drug. Hence the result of "dechallenge" is meaningless. This type of reaction may be coded as "possible".*
>
> *4.3.7.2. Stroke. Some patients recover fully, some partially, some remain severely disabled and some die. All these outcomes are part of the natural history of the disease and, with very few exceptions, are unrelated to drug withdrawal. Again, the result*

of "dechallenge" is usually meaningless. This type of reaction may be coded as "possible".

4.3.7.3. Acute anaphylaxis immediately following an injection. Here there is an obvious direct relationship, but the usual parameters for establishing relationship, e.g. dechallenge do not apply. In this example, the best category for the relationship is "certain".

4.4. Unlikely

4.4.1. The event occurred with a duration to onset that makes a causal effect improbable with the drug being considered. (The pharmacology of the drug and nature of the event should be considered in arriving at this conclusion.)

4.4.2. The event commenced before the first administration of the drug.

4.4.3. The drug was withdrawn and this made no difference to the event when, clinically, recovery would be expected. (This would not apply for some serious events such as myocardial infarction, or events causing permanent damage.)

4.4.4. It is strongly suggestive of a non-causal relationship if the drug was continued and the event resolved.

4.5. Unclassified or conditional

These are reports with insufficient data to establish a relationship and more data are expected. This is a temporary repository, and the category for these events will be finalized when the new data become available.

4.6. Unassessable

4.6.1. An event has occurred in association with a drug, but there is insufficient data to make an assessment.

4.6.2. Some of the data may be contradictory or inconsistent.

4.6.3. Details of the report cannot be supplemented or verified.

5. Processes for establishing the relationship

To ensure a methodical approach to relationship assessment, the use of the coding sheet referred to in section E.3.4 is very helpful. (See Annex 2 for an example). The following should be recorded systematically before data entry:

5.1. Result of dechallenge

Select the most appropriate outcome:

5.1.1. recovered;

5.1.2. improved;

5.1.3. no change;

5.1.4. worse;

5.1.5. don't know;

5.1.6. no dechallenge (medicine continued).

5.2. Result of rechallenge with the same medicine by itself

Select the most appropriate outcome:

5.2.1. recurrence of problem;

5.2.2. no recurrence;

5.2.3. don't know;

5.2.4. no rechallenge.

5.3. Outcome of the event

Select the most appropriate term:

5.3.1. recovered;

5.3.2. improving (as at a recorded date);

5.3.3. died;

5.3.4. permanent disability;

5.3.5. unknown.

5.4. Clinical details

5.4.1. Concomitant disease.

5.4.2. Relevant patient history, e.g. liver disease; renal disease.

5.4.3. Previous exposure to same medicine(s).

5.4.3.1. Yes/no?

5.4.3.2. Any reaction to previous exposure – yes/no.

5.4.3.3. If "yes", record the reaction term(s) for previous reaction(s).

5.5. Logic check

It is very easy to make mistakes in assigning a relationship. The final step should be a check on your logic. Some of the considerations are as follows:

5.5.1. You should not have a relationship of "certain" if there has been no rechallenge, or the outcome of rechallenge is unknown.

5.5.2. You should not have a relationship of "probable" if there has been no dechallenge or the result of dechallenge is unknown.

5.5.3. You should not have a relationship of "probable" if the outcome of the event is unknown.

5.5.4. You should not have a relationship of "probable" if there are other possible causes of the event.

H. Signal identification

(from spontaneous reports or cohort event monitoring)

1. Introduction

1.1. General approach

The identification of signals in the National Centre's database requires careful review of individual reports and events. Careful, informed, routine, systematic and standardized clinical review of the Centre's reports with the recording and appropriate collation of good data provides the quickest and most satisfying way of identifying previously unsuspected adverse reactions. Following through the whole process from relationship assessment, to signal identification, to signal strengthening, to communicating the findings is essential.

1.2. Definition of a signal

1.2.1. "Reported information on a possible causal relationship between an adverse event and a drug, the relationship being unknown or incompletely documented previously."

1.2.2. Alternatively, there are several events (or sometimes a single event) with a strong relationship ("certain" or "probable" and sometimes "possible") and there does not seem to be good evidence anywhere of it being recognized as a reaction.

1.2.3. There may be one or two case-reports in the literature, but this is insufficient as validation and the signal needs to be strengthened.

1.3. Reference sources on adverse reactions

1.3.1. Martindale. The Complete Drug Reference is probably the most reliable source.

1.3.2. The Physicians Desk Reference (PDR) is also useful. However, the entries are mainly data sheets provided by pharmaceutical companies and contain many references to possible reactions that are not validated and the information is often difficult to interpret.

1.3.3. Micromedex online drug reference is a reliable reference.

1.3.4. If there is not good evidence of an event being recognized as an adverse reaction in two or more of these references, then, if warranted clinically, it should be investigated further as a possible signal.

2. Good data are essential

2.1. The data in the report(s) need to be of good quality if a signal of a new adverse reaction is to be considered.

2.2. There should be sufficient data to fully assess the relationship of the drug to the event. The strongest signals will have several reports with a "certain" or "probable" relationship. A signal may be possible from one very good "certain" report. If there are no "certain" reports, at least three "probable" reports would be necessary for a signal.

2.3. The first reports with a "certain" or "probable" relationship are called "index cases".

2.4. Cases with a "possible" relationship can only provide supporting evidence. A group of unexpected deaths coded as "possible" forms an exception to this general rule and will need to be taken seriously.

2.5. Cases coded as "unclassified" or "unassessable" should not be considered in the investigation of a signal.

2.6. A group of "unlikely" reports may sometimes produce a signal of an unexpected reaction. However, they should not be included in the assessment of a signal for which there are reports with certain, probable or possible relationships because they are different and could mask the characteristics of the signal being investigated.

3. Selection criteria for events to investigate

3.1. There are good data.

3.2. The event is clinically relevant.

3.3. There have been several reports of the event that show a credible and strong relationship with the drug (certain or probable).

3.4. If validated, the event is of sufficient importance or interest to:

3.4.1. require regulatory action;

3.4.2. require advice to prescribers;

3.4.3. be of scientific importance.

4. Methods of signal identification

- clinical assessment of individual events
- clinical review of collated events
- record linkage
- automated signal detection.

4.1. Clinical assessment of individual events

4.1.1. Careful, routine, standardized clinical assessment of individual reports, as described in section G, with alertness to the possibility of a signal, offers the quickest method of identifying signals.

4.1.2. This approach should be taken during routine review of incoming reports.

4.1.2.1. During routine assessment of reports, if an assessor identifies an event and thinks that it could be a new type of adverse reaction, a search should be undertaken for records of other similar events to confirm the opinion.

4.1.2.2. First check the adverse reaction reference sources (section I.1.3).

4.1.2.3. If there is no reference to the occurrence of the event as an adverse reaction, proceed with its investigation.

4.2. Clinical review of collated events

4.2.1. All the events in the database for the drug of interest (or class of drugs) should be reviewed at regular intervals e.g. each month.

4.2.2. This is facilitated by collating (sorting) the events using a clinically orientated structure. This is accomplished by sorting on the events dictionary print codes (see section D.9.3.).

4.2.3. Collating the events.

4.2.3.1. By this stage, the individual events have been assessed, and each event should have had a term applied to it that is selected from the events dictionary. There is a dictionary code for each of these terms and this should be added to the database with the terms during data entry.

4.2.3.2. The dictionary terms should be coded in such a way that clinically related events appear together when the events are sorted by the code.

4.2.3.3. The events can then be printed out or seen on the computer monitor in the desired clinical structure. Groups of related events can then be seen clearly.

4.2.3.4. Example: For the investigation of cardiac failure as a possible signal, all possibly related events, and conditions that may be associated with heart failure, should be grouped together. These would include cardiac failure aggravated, cardiac failure right, congestive heart failure, cardiac failure left, dyspnoea (in the absence of respiratory disease), peripheral oedema, cardiomegaly, cardiomyopathy and heart valve disorders. The whole group of events should then be taken into consideration. (See Annex 5 for such an events collation.)

4.2.3.5. WHO-ART is easily adapted for coding in this way and additional terms can be added for the event monitoring.

4.2.3.6. Annex 9 is a table which illustrates the collation of events in a clinical hierarchy and which also shows a signal.

- *The table shows eye events reported as being associated with COX-2 inhibitors from the IMMP in New Zealand*

- *The IMMP dictionary code can be seen in the column headed "PRTCODE".*

- *The column headed "REL" is the relationship column: 1 = certain; 2 = probable; 3 = possible; 4 =*

unlikely; 5 = unclassified; 6 = unassessable. In this way, the strength of the relationship can be seen as well as the number of occurrences of each event.

• The listing demonstrates a signal of disturbance of vision including temporary blindness and visual field defect. All but one of the events listed under "Visual–Acuity" form part of the signal. There is one report that is "certain" and 12 "probable" reports. That makes a strong signal. There were four reports with a "possible" relationship which give supporting evidence. There was also one report that is "unlikely" because there was another cause for the event. The reports under "Disturbance" are also likely to be related to this signal.

• This signal was published and is a good illustration of how to develop and validate a signal. (Coulter DM, Clark DWJ. Disturbance of vision by COX-2 inhibitors. *Expert Opinion on Drug Safety, 2004, 3:607–614.)*

4.2.4. Special types of event

4.2.4.1. Deaths should be entered with the cause(s) given. Death in itself is an event and deaths are best listed in a separate Clinical Category. The causes of death should be collated within this Category in the same way as events generally, using the dictionary code, so that they appear in clinically meaningful groupings. Any clinical patterns associated with death can then be seen easily. Rigorous validation procedures should then be applied to any suspicious patterns forming a signal (see section I). An example of a collated listing of deaths is shown in Annex 8.

4.2.4.2. Signals of interactions: Potential interactions should also be listed in a separate Clinical Category called "Associations" for ease of signal identification. This Category is called "Associations" because it is a listing of potential interactions only. It is a record of events occurring with more than one medicine used. The concomitant medicines should be listed with the events that occurred. An example of a listing of Associations is shown in Annex 10.

4.2.5. Review of events coded "unlikely".

4.2.5.1. There is always the possibility that unexpected reactions have been coded as "unlikely" and represent missed signals.

4.2.5.2. These events should be examined regularly for any unexpected patterns. If unexpected patterns emerge, they should be treated as signals and investigated as in section I.

4.3. Record linkage

4.3.1. Record linkage depends on the availability of a unique identifier for patients in the health system or in hospital records.

4.3.2. This same identifier must also be recorded with the patient details in the cohort database.

4.3.3. It can then be used as a tool to gather additional events data for the cohort, particularly on events that occur after the follow-up.

4.3.4. The process involves matching the patient identifiers in the cohort with patients that have the same identifier in any available databases or registers (e.g. register of deaths or hospital admissions).

4.3.5. When the patient records are linked in this way, it is possible to see, for example:

4.3.5.1. if the patient has died and the date and cause of death;

4.3.5.2. if the patient has been admitted to hospital and the diagnoses;

4.3.5.3. if the patient has been diagnosed with a disease of special interest for which a register has been created.

4.3.6. The results of the linkage are then reviewed and added to the records of events for the patients in the cohort. An unexpectedly high rate of a particular event (e.g. dystonic reactions or liver damage identified from hospital discharge diagnoses), may represent a signal.

4.3.7. Methods

4.3.7.1. The Uppsala Monitoring Centre UMC) regularly scans the WHO database for potential signals using its automated data mining programme the Bayesian Confidence Propagation Neural Network (BCPNN). This produces Information Component (IC) values for drug–event combinations. These can be plotted as graphs over time to examine any trend. A positive signal will have IC values that become more significant over time as more cases are included. This represents worldwide experience in the world's largest database.

4.3.7.2. The UMC will run this programme on request to investigate a particular drug–event combination of interest to your centre.

4.3.7.3. Proportional reporting ratios (PRR). This is a method that uses software to measure the proportion of reports in the database with a particular drug–event combination and compares this proportion with that for the same event in the reports for all other drugs combined. If the PRR for a particular drug–event combination is significantly high, it may represent a signal.

4.3.8. Usefulness

4.3.8.1. Automated methods can strengthen a signal identified by clinical evaluation.

4.3.8.2. They may identify signals that were missed during assessment of the reports and later review.

4.3.8.3. The BCPNN runs on all reported events worldwide and there is therefore a greater chance of finding more reports of the suspect drug–event combination. It is performed on a routine basis.

5. Comment

5.1. Identifying signals in "real time" by clinical evaluation during routine assessment and regular review of the events in the database for a drug, will find most signals earlier than automated methods.

5.2. PRR methods are more reliable in large databases, but are still somewhat experimental and lack reliability.

5.3. All signals identified from statistical programmes (BCPNN or PRR) require subsequent clinical evaluation.

I. Strengthening the signal

1. General approach

Clinical evaluation of signals identified by the BCPNN may also be thought of as "strengthening" the signal because conclusions reached from the process of "validating" a signal are often not final. The signal may however be strengthened with the further evidence gained. The process entails examining other available data and also examining your own data in greater depth according to the following principles:

1.1. reviewing other experience;

1.2. searching for non-random patterns;

1.3. reviewing the pharmacology;

1.4. consulting your expert safety review panel and other experts;

1.5. undertaking epidemiological studies;

1.6. communication and feedback.

2. Other experience

2.1. Are there other similar reports in the Centre's database? Look for *related clinical events* for the suspect drug. Also, look at *related drugs* in the same ATC classification grouping.

2.2. Search the worldwide database of suspected adverse reactions of the WHO Collaborating Centre (the Uppsala Monitoring Centre, available at: https://vigisearch.who-umc.org/).

2.3. Request the Information Component (IC) value for the drug–event combination from the WHO Collaborating Centre (the Uppsala Monitoring Centre). (This will indicate if the particular drug–event combination has been reported more often than would be expected and give a measure of the statistical significance.) The IC value for a drug–event combination can often be found in the combinations database provided to National Centres by the UMC.

2.4. Ask for information held by other National Centres through the Vigimed email network coordinated by the UMC.

2.5. Search the literature for similar reports, using search tools such as PubMed or Micromedex.

2.6. Ask the pharmaceutical company if they have received similar reports and ask for details.

2.7. Were similar events identified in clinical trials? (Search the literature for reports of clinical trials of the medicine.)

2.8. Were similar events identified in preclinical studies? (Ask the pharmaceutical company.)

2.9. Has this event or have any similar events been identified in postmarketing cohort event monitoring (prescription event monitoring or IMMP) studies?

3. Search for non-random patterns

Examination of data on a group of reports may show patterns that are not random and, in the absence of biases, non-random patterns suggest that the events may be related to the medicine.

3.1. Onset times: Does the range of onset times cluster around a particular period (e.g. 5 days or 3 weeks), or are the onset times scattered randomly over time? Compare the onset times of the cases with those for the rest of the cohort using life-table or survival analysis.)

3.2. Is the mean dose significantly higher in those who experienced the event being studied than in those in whom the event did not occur?

3.3. Is the mean age of patients in whom the event occured significantly different from that of those who did not experience the event?

3.4. Sex differences: when compared with the cohort, are the rates of the event in men and women significantly different?

4. Pharmacology

4.1. Is there a plausible pharmacological mechanism by which the drug could cause the event?

4.2. Have other drugs in the same class caused a similar problem and has a mechanism been described for the related drug(s)?

4.3. Note that with a new medicine there may not be a known

mechanism for a new adverse reaction. Sometimes the study of a previously unidentified adverse reaction brings to light new knowledge about the pharmacology of the medicine.

5. Investigative epidemiological studies

Investigative epidemiological studies may be needed if the event seems important. These studies may require collaboration with others who have expertise in this field. Such studies include:

5.1. cohort studies;

5.2. case–control studies;

5.3. record linkage studies;

5.4. population database studies.

6. Communication

Effective, well-presented communication of the signal to the various stakeholders will inform and give you feedback on its validity and its importance. The following stakeholders can provide invaluable advice:

6.1. Expert Safety Review Panel and/or regulatory authority;

6.2. health practitioners;

6.3. The Uppsala Monitoring Centre;

6.4. the pharmaceutical company;

6.5. country ADR bulletin;

6.6. letter or report to a medical journal.

J. Identifying risk factors

1. Introduction

1.1. Definition

1.1.1. A risk factor is a characteristic associated with an increased probability of occurrence of an event . In the presence of a risk factor, a patient is more likely to develop an adverse reaction. Knowledge of risk factors provides a means of avoiding or minimizing the adverse reactions they relate to. Risk factors may be associated with:

1.1.1.1. the patient;

1.1.1.2. the medicine;

1.1.1.3. the environment.

1.2. Risk factors associated with the patient

1.2.1. age

1.2.2. size: weight and height or body mass index (BMI)

1.2.3. genetic polymorphism (CYP 450 enzymes)

1.2.4. ethnicity (e.g. G6PD and primaquine)

1.2.5. pregnancy

1.2.6. concomitant illness (e.g. HIV/AIDS)

1.2.7. renal or liver damage.

1.3. Risk factors linked to the medicine

1.3.1. dose

1.3.2. duration of therapy

1.3.3. previous exposure (allergic type reactions)

1.3.4. concomitant medicines.

1.4. Risk factors linked to the culture or environment

1.4.1. cigarette smoking

1.4.2. alcohol or other drugs

1.4.3. diet (e.g. grapefruit juice).

2. Identification

2.1. Pharmacology

Knowledge of the pharmacodynamics and pharmacokinetics of a drug may allow certain adverse reactions to be predicted, but does not identify them.

2.2. Clinical trials

Risk factors for certain adverse reactions might be identified in clinical trials, but these trials are not designed to examine safety issues and the opportunity is limited because of small numbers of participants.

2.3. Clinical experience

Clinical experience might create the impression that certain characteristics are risk factors, but if rates are not measured, these impressions are unreliable.

2.4. Spontaneous reporting

2.4.1. Risk factors cannot be identified with certainty from spontaneous reporting because of the absence of rates. If a particular characteristic appears more frequently than expected in adverse reaction reports e.g. younger age group, it might be assumed that this is a risk factor, but such assumptions are unreliable.

2.4.2. Rates can be calculated using the defined daily dose (DDD), but these estimates suffer from the fact that spontaneous reporting is incomplete and the rates will be very low. Also there are often strong biases in spontaneous reporting which distort the findings. However, rates based on DDDs can be useful for comparing similar medicines given under similar conditions if every effort is made to identify possible confounders.

2.5. Cohort event monitoring

2.5.1. With knowledge of the characteristics of the whole cohort it is possible to measure the differences between patients in whom adverse reactions occur and those in whom they do not and thus identify risk factors.

2.5.2. The simplest approach is to measure the relative risk (RR) of a characteristic in patients from the cohort who have experienced the adverse reaction under investigation, compared with patients in the cohort in whom the reaction did not occur. The RR is calculated by dividing the rate in those who did have the reaction by the rate in those who did not have the reaction. In practice it is the proportion of patients with the suspected risk factor taking the medicine and who have had the reaction divided by the proportion of patients with the suspected risk factor taking the medicine, who did not have the reaction under investigation. Confidence intervals (CI) should be calculated in order to assess the statistical significance of any difference found. This method is subject to biases or confounders because of possible differences between the two groups e.g. concomitant medicines or prescribing bias. These differences might be multiple e.g. concomitant disease plus cigarette smoking.

2.5.3. Multiple logistic regression is a powerful statistical method that will control for several characteristics in the one calculation and identify risk factors reliably. If you wish to employ this method it is best to consult a biostatistician.

2.5.4. Case–control studies can be undertaken to examine characteristics for which no data has been collected. As an example, abnormal renal function might be suspected as a risk factor. To investigate this, a sample of patients who have had the adverse reaction under investigation is selected together with a matching sample of patients in the cohort who did not have the adverse reaction. Renal function tests are then undertaken and the rates of abnormal function calculated for each group. The RR of abnormal renal function in the reaction group compared with those who did not have the reaction is then calculated. Confidence intervals for the RR will reveal whether any difference found is statistically significant and if abnormal renal function is a risk factor. (This is called a "nested" case–control study".)

K. Analyses

A number of different analyses have been mentioned in this manual. All but one or two can be undertaken by pharmacovigilance staff. Some statistical software is available online e.g. MedCalc. This allows 25 free analyses, but then requires a payment for continued use. It is not expensive. However, it is hoped that all the required functions will be made available in the VigiFlow adaptation for CEM. Not all of these methods are applicable to spontaneous reporting.

This section is mainly a listing in two categories of the analytical methods that are likely to be most helpful: data manipulation and statistical methods.

1. Data manipulation

1.1. Tabular

1.1.1. summary of reporting rates for males, females and totals;

1.1.2. age/sex profiles of the cohort;

1.1.3. patient numbers by region;

1.1.4. event profiles by clinical category;

1.1.5. clinically oriented listing of events with sex, age, dose, duration to onset, relationship, and outcome. This tabulation gives a very good clinical picture of the events occurring in the cohort (see Annex 5);

1.1.6. comparison of event profiles pretreatment and post-treatment;

1.1.7. rates of important events pretreatment and post-treatment with relative risks;

1.1.8. table of the most frequent post-treatment events with numbers and rates and outcome (treatment withdrawn, deaths);

1.1.9. case-report listing (lists all events for each case-report);

1.1.10. reasons for withdrawal of treatment.

1.2. Graphic

Some of the above information (e.g. the profiles) can be presented helpfully as bar graph (see Annex 6).

2. Statistical analyses

2.1. Relative risk (RR) with confidence intervals (CI).

2.2. *t test* for the comparison of means.

2.3. Life-table analysis (survival analysis). For the event being studied, this type of analysis identifies the duration to onset for every patient who experienced the event and calculates the rates for patients in whom the event has occurred (or the survivors) at specified points in time. This can be used to measure the range of onset times of any event and to assess if there is a non-random relationship with the drug (see section I.3.3.1.).

2.4. Multiple logistic regression. This is used mainly for determining risk factors. This type of analysis should be undertaken only by a biostatistician.

L. Differences between spontaneous reporting and cohort event monitoring

1. Cohort event monitoring

1.1. Advantages

1.1.1. the ability to produce rates;

1.1.2. the ability to produce a near complete profile of the adverse event and/or adverse reaction for the medicines of interest;

1.1.3. very effective in identifying signals at an early stage;

1.1.4. the ability to characterize reactions in terms of age, sex and duration to onset and thus produce risk factors. Other relevant data may be collected such as weight, or comorbidity in order to provide the opportunity for determining other risk factors;

1.1.5. the ability to make accurate comparisons between medicines;

1.1.6. the ability to establish a pregnancy register and define and measure rates of any abnormalities;

1.1.7. because of the routine follow-up, the method can detect with confidence reduced or failed therapeutic effect and thus raise suspicion of inaccurate diagnosis of disease, poor prescribing, inadequate adherence to treatment, emerging resistance or poor quality or counterfeit medicines;

1.1.8. the ability to record and examine details of all deaths and provide rates of death;

1.1.9. the ability to produce rapid results in a defined population;

1.1.10. this method collects comprehensive and near-complete data that will provide for the special needs of the malaria programme, including effects of malaria treatment in pregnancy, specific toxicities, safety in children;

1.1.11. because the method looks intensively at new drugs of great interest in a specific area of need, and provides clinically significant results rapidly, it stimulates interest in drug safety in general;

1.1.12. the method provides sound evidence with which to deal with any drug scares.

1.2. Disadvantages

1.2.1. The method is more labour intensive and more costly than spontaneous reporting.

1.2.2. It will be new to health professionals and Pharmacovigilance Centres and training in its use will be necessary.

2. Spontaneous reporting

2.1. Advantages

2.1.1. It is administratively simpler and less labour intensive than CEM.

2.1.2. It is less costly than CEM.

2.1.3. It is the most common method of pharmacovigilance used.

2.1.4. National Pharmacovigilance Centres and health professionals (to a certain extent) will be familiar with this method.

2.2. Disadvantages

2.2.1. The data collected by this method are incomplete. In developed countries less than 5% of reactions are reported. A report from the WHO filariasis programme suggests that compliance with reporting is likely to be much lower than this, leaving many unanswered questions.

2.2.2. Reliable rates cannot be calculated and so risk cannot be measured and risk factors cannot be established with confidence.

2.2.3. There are strong biases in reporting.

2.2.4. Deaths are poorly reported.

2.2.5. Special studies will need to be set up to obtain accurate information on areas of particular interest e.g. pregnancy, children and specific events of concern. These special studies add to the cost and in turn reduce the cost advantage of spontaneous reporting.

M. Organization

1. Legislation

1.1. Legal authorization

Spontaneous reporting and CEM programmes form the data collection arms of pharmacovigilance activities. The collection of data required for spontaneous reporting and CEM programmes should be authorized or required by law. Pharmacovigilance is non-interventional and will not create any physical risk to patients. Spontaneous reporting and CEM programmes are not clinical trials. They are methods of public health surveillance requiring the collection of certain types of data in the public interest. Public health surveillance is frequently conducted under specific laws authorizing or requiring the collection of certain types of data. In some countries, reporting on the risks associated with medicines is mandatory. All medicines are subject to spontaneous reporting. Selected new medicines that are to be used widely and are of public health importance should be subject to CEM where possible. The ACT antimalarials are typical examples of such medicines. Leaders in the field of pharmacovigilance in each country should advocate the legal endorsement or requirement for pharmacovigilance activities of both types.

1.2. Conditional registration

The legal status of pharmacovigilance data collection can be reinforced by further legal requirements or regulations that require specified new medicines of public health importance to be subject to CEM before full registration is granted. Conditional registration can be offered until the outcome of a CEM study is known, at which time full registration can be approved or declined on the grounds of safety.

1.3. Regulation of professional standards

In many countries the standards of health professionals are maintained and improved by compulsory continuing medical education (CME). It is justifiable for CME credits to be given for pharmacovigilance activities. Sending spontaneous reports or CEM questionnaires to the Pharmacovigilance Centre displays, on the part of the health professional concerned, professional responsibility, good medical practice and involvement in activities that improve the standard of patient care and safety. In addition, the activity provides a learning process both through the completion of the forms, which requires thinking about safety issues, and from the feedback received from the Pharmacovigilance Centre. Professional associations should be encouraged to include spontaneous reporting and CEM in their approved CME activities.

2. Ethical issues

2.1. Introduction

2.1.1. Ethical principles must be applied consistently to all types of pharmacovigilance methods. The ethics of collecting data for CEM, in particular, have special features since it is a methodology which requires the collection of detailed personal data and sometimes stores these data for indefinite periods. There may often be a need for follow-up at a later date for the further study of any safety concerns identified, at which time there will be a need to conduct investigations such as a more detailed cohort study, nested case–control studies, comparative safety studies, subgroup investigations (e.g. in children) or even a full clinical trial.

2.1.2. Before starting the process of commencing a CEM programme, there must be open discussions with all the stakeholders including patients, the general public and community leaders, all health providers, professional organizations, the pharmaceutical industry, the media and, finally, the health ministry and politicians without whose support little will be achieved.

2.1.3. The security, privacy and confidentiality of personal data need to be strenuously maintained, because it is essential to record personal identifiers. Pharmacovigilance will not work properly if personal identifiers are not available. With both spontaneous reporting and CEM programmes, the ability to follow up specific patients on important outcomes is essential. With CEM, which can measure risk (incidence) and identify risk factors, it is essential that duplicate entries are avoided so that the accuracy of these findings is not compromised, and this can only be done if patients can be correctly identified. This necessity for recording patient identifiers therefore imposes strict conditions on maintaining data security. These are outlined as follows:

2.2. Prerequisites to collecting patient data

2.2.1. It is important to seek the approval of the highest appropriate authority in the country. This may be the ministry of health or the regulatory authority.

2.2.2. It is important to declare publicly what data are being collected and why.

2.2.3. The stated purposes should be broad enough to include:

> *2.2.3.1. long-term follow-up looking for signals of delayed reactions;*
>
> *2.2.3.2. use of the data to enable follow-up investigations such as nested case–control studies to be undertaken to identify risk factors. It is not always possible to predict what additional studies might be needed for the investigation of safety issues that are identified during monitoring;*
>
> *2.2.3.3. follow-up studies required to validate signals;*
>
> *2.2.3.4. comparative studies with new antimalarials.*

2.2.4. Security and confidentiality arrangements should be

publicized and should conform with any national legislative requirements.

2.3 Training of staff

2.3.1. Staff members responsible for pharmacovigilance need to be trained in the strict maintenance of security and confidentiality.

2.3.2. They should be required to sign a document saying that they understand the privacy issues and have been taught how to agree to maintain security and confidentiality.

2.4. Security issues

2.4.1. Data that might identify patients should be stored on computers with no Internet link. This prevents access by hackers. This precaution will be impractical and unnecessary for those using VigiFlow and its CEM adaptation.

2.4.2. Access to a computer that has data on it that might identify patients should be controlled by password.

2.4.3. Password access should be given only to those people involved in the particular pharmacovigilance activity.

2.4.4. Access to the premises should be security controlled.

2.5. Use of data

2.5.1. The data collected should be used only for the purposes declared.

2.5.2. Personal identifiable data should not be given to any other parties including pharmaceutical companies, government or ministry officials, agencies and research groups. This includes personal details of patients or reporters.

2.6. Confidentiality

2.6.1. No published data, including reports, should contain any information that could identify patients.

2.6.2. Staff should not take any identifiable data home or to other places outside the Pharmacovigilance Centre.

2.6.3. Staff should not discuss information outside the Pharmacovigilance Centre that could lead to the identification of any patient.

2.7. Informed consent

2.7.1. If pharmacovigilance activities, spontaneous reports and CEM, are authorized or required by law, informed consent from individual patients is not required for the collection of data required for safety monitoring. However all the privacy conditions outlined above should be strictly observed.

2.7.2. Programme managers should avoid attempting to obtain individual informed consent if at all possible because it will be time-consuming to try to explain the concepts of pharmacovigilance (which will often be culturally strange) to each patient, will increase complexity and add to the cost, and could potentially compromise the validity of the results if many patients refuse to be enrolled. A CEM programme is **not** a clinical trial and does not interfere with treatment in any way. It is simply a process of data collection.

2.7.3. An alternative to obtaining informed consent from individual patients is to provide information publicly (see section D.3) and to give patients leaflets which they can study, or have explained to them, away from the pressure of the clinics, and which provide them with contact details for the health facility and Pharmacovigilance Centre so that they can object to having their data stored if this is their decision. Their data can then not be entered or if they have already been entered, they will be deleted. This is called the "opt out principle" which operates in a number of countries and, if needed, is much more practical than individual informed consent.

3. Structure

3.1. The development of a Pharmacovigilance Centre and its relationship to public health programmes is discussed fully in the following WHO publications:

3.1.1. Safety monitoring of medicinal products: Guidelines for setting up and running a Pharmacovigilance Centre. WHO 2000

3.1.2. The safety of medicines in public health programmes: Pharmacovigilance an essential tool. WHO 2006

3.2. Centre staff

3.2.1. It is essential that the Pharmacovigilance Centre has sufficient additional capacity to run CEM studies. For two parallel CEM studies (ie a comparator study of two antimalarials) to be undertaken, it is suggested that the following personnel would be necessary:

3.2.2. A full-time clinical supervisor who would be in charge of the CEM activities. This person would:

> *3.2.2.1. Review the events reported on the questionnaires and would undertake relationship assessment, arrange follow-up of reports as required, liaise with the malaria programme manager, request appropriate data analysis, report regularly to the Expert Safety Review Panel in conjunction with the malaria programme manager and consult them about any concerns arising from the data, any reports of serious events and any signals of new adverse reactions.*
>
> *3.2.2.2. Be responsible for communication in collaboration with the malaria programme manager. This would involve promotional activities as outlined in section D.3.*
>
> *3.2.2.3. Be responsible for the training of Centre and peripheral staff.*

3.2.3. A full-time data manager. This person would maintain the database, be responsible for quality assurance, ensure security and confidentiality of data, be responsible for collating the data and producing reports as required, ensure the supply of questionnaires to all health facilities, train and supervise the data processor and generally assist the clinical supervisor.

3.2.4. One full-time data processor employed for the duration of the monitoring programme. This person would be responsible for data entry and certain other tasks under the supervision of the data manager.

3.3. Peripheral staff

3.3.1. The peripheral staff will be under the supervision of a person with the role of field coordinator who will be responsible to the malaria programme manager and the clinical supervisor of the CEM studies. A simple chain of responsibility will need to be planned.

3.3.2. Staff from the malaria programme (MP) or the Sentinel Site (SS) or the national Pharmacovigilance Centre will need to be available:

3.3.2.1. To facilitate in every way possible the collection of the data required for the CEM study (MP).

3.3.2.2. To ensure delivery and collection of questionnaires (MP).

3.3.2.3. To maintain a local register of patients included in the CEM activity, to ensure appointments are made for a follow-up visit to the health facility and to undertake follow-up of patients who miss their return appointment (SS).

3.3.2.4. To ensure follow-up of women who are known to be pregnant, and any women of child-bearing age, if they miss their follow-up visit to the health facility where they were treated. They will also need to liaise with antenatal clinics and birthing facilities to collect follow-up data on the pregnancy and the outcome of childbirth (SS).

3.3.2.5. To ensure follow-up of all deaths in order to find out the history of events leading to death, the cause of death and the date of death (Pharmacovigilance Centre).

N. Communication

Good communication is imperative at all times and its importance has been highlighted throughout this manual. Some basic principles are described in Annex 14. As described in this manual, essential aspects of communication embrace two main objectives:

- promotion or advocacy of the methodology;
- sharing the results.

Communication is a two-way process, which means the Pharmacovigilance Centre should listen to and carefully consider the opinions of others. Much can be learnt and much goodwill can be created from this process even if you cannot accept or implement all the suggestions that are made.

The following groups need to be included in the communication process:

- patients and the general public;
- all players involved in the supply and therapeutic management of malaria;
- those with regulatory and public health responsibilities;
- the appropriate government officials;
- the appropriate academic institutions and departments;
- relevant professional organizations including the opinion leaders and practitioners;
- international: WHO including regional offices, the UMC and VigiMed;
- the media;
- staff of the Pharmacovigilance Centre, the Expert Safety Review Panel and others involved in the activities of monitoring.

See the following sections for specific references:

D.3; D.7; I.6; M.2.2.2.2.

O. Annexes

(*Listed in order of reference in the text*)

1. CEM reporting form sides A and B.
2. Coding sheet.
3. Clinical Categories in IMMP events dictionary.
4. Clinical Category Eyes IMMP events dictionary.
5. Sample events collation, IMMP, omeprazole, Circulatory.
6. Sample comparative events profiles, IMMP, celecoxib and rofecoxib.
7. CEM pregnancy questionnaire.
8. Sample listing of deaths as events, IMMP, omeprazole.
9. Eye events collation demonstrating a signal, IMMP.
10. Sample listing of drug-drug associations for celecoxib, IMMP.
11. A selection of helpful websites.
12. References.
13. Contacts.
14. Some basic principles of communication.

Annex I - Adverse Event Report Form - ACT Cohort Event Monitoring

Pre-treatment Questionnaire - Side A

Health facility: ....

1. Patient Details:

First name: ....Family name.................. Patient Identification Number..................
Date of birth: ..../..../.... Age: .....years; for children<1 year:.....months
Gender: Male□ Female □ Weight (kg): ....Height (cm): ....
Pregnant: No□ Uncertain□ Yes □ if yes specify: 1st □ 2nd □ 3rd □ trimester
Address: ....
Nearest contact person for patient follow-up: ....

2. Signs and symptoms at presentation:

....
....

3. Malaria laboratory tests results *(Blank row is for additional tests)*

Test	Date	Result	Test	Date	Result
Microscopy	..../..../....		Rapid Diagnostic Test	..../..../....	
Hb/Ht level	..../..../....				

4. Medicines taken during previous two weeks

Name of medicine	Indication	Dose & frequency	Date started	Date stopped [1]
			..../..../....	..../..../....
			..../..../....	..../..../....
			..../..../....	..../..../....

4.1 Traditional herbal medicines taken during previous two weeks: No□ Yes □

5. All clinical events in the last 5 days

Conditions	Date

6. Present or past medical conditions

Conditions	Present	Past

[1] If the treatment continues during the study period, write under this column "continue"

7. Medicines prescribed at this visit

Name	Dose & Frequency	Date started	Expected completion
ACT (specify brand)		…./…./….	…./…./….
		…./…./….	…./…./….
		…./…./….	…./…./….

8. Date of planned follow-up visit in health facility: …./…./…

9.Reporter:

Name……………………………….Signature:…………………………Date…/…/…..
Cell. Phone number …………………………….

Post-treatment Questionnaire - Side B

10. Type of follow-up

Attendance at health center / clinic ☐ Date …./…./….
Visit at home ☐ Date …./…./….
Other (specify) ……………………………….. Date …./…./….
Follow-up visit at home by: Name………………………………..Signature:……………………

11. All medicines taken at any time during ACT treatment (days 0-3)

Name	Indication	Dose & frequency	Date started	Date stopped
ACT (specify brand)			…./…./….	…./…./….
			…./…./….	…./…./….
			…./…./….	…./…./….

12. Outcomes noted at post-treatment visit

Outcome	Tick	Outcome	Tick
Adhered to complete treatment		Incomplete adherence to treatment	
Improvement of clinical condition		Deterioration of clinical condition	
No change in clinical condition		New clinical event	
No referral to health center/hospital		Referral to health center/hospital	
Lost to follow-up		Reasons for referral:	

13. In case of incomplete adherence to ACT treatment

Record reasons given by patient or caretaker for not completing treatment as prescribed

14. Describe new events or worsening problems after starting ACT treatment

Description of event	Date event started	Date event stopped	Suspect Medicine	Outcome * (A,B,C etc)
1.	…./…./….	…./…./….		
2.	…./…./….	…./…./….		
3.	…./…./….	…./…./….		

* Outcome: A - recovered B - improved C - unchanged D - life threatening
E - caused or prolonged hospitalization F - persistent incapacity or disability
G - death (date …./…./….) O - Other (describe)
………………….................

15. Abnormal laboratory tests results after starting ACT treatment

Test	Date	Result	Test	Date	Result
	…./…./….			…./…./….	

16.Reporter:

Name……………………………….Signature:………………………………Date…/…/…..

Mobile phone number ……………………

PLEASE SEND THIS FORM TO:

…………………………………………………………………………………………

……………………………………………………………………………………

The report should be sent immediately if the outcome of the adverse event is: death, life-threatening, persistent incapacity or disability, caused or prolonged hospitalization.

Please note: ***Completion of this form is not an admission of causation by, or contribution to, the suspected adverse event by the suspected medicine(s) or by the reporting professionals. This information will be analysed and will contribute to promoting the safe use of antimalarials.***

Annex 2. Coding sheet – sample from the IMMP[1]

NAME | SOURCE | REPORT NO

Monitored Medicine

Dose | Indication

	Event	Sev	Rel	Pnt	Duration Onset	Duration Event
1						
2						
3						
4						
5						

Outcome

- A Recovered without seq
- B Recovered with seq
- F Not yet recovered
- D Died - due to AR
- C Died - med may be contributory
- N Died - unrelated to med
- O Died - cause unknown
- U Unknown

Seriousness

Dechallenge

1. Definite improvement
2. No improvement
3. Med continued
4. Unknown

Rechallenge

1. Recurrence
2. No recurrence
3. No rechallenge
4. Unknown

Category

Dose Reduced | **Withdrawn** | **Died**

Abbreviations:

Sev = severity

Rel = relationship

Pnt = print-code

'Category' refers to the major Clinical Category in which the event should be classified.

[1] Intensive Medicines Monitoring Programme.

Annex 3. Major Clinical Categories IMMP Events Dictionary[1]

1. Accidents
2. Alimentary
3. Autonomic
4. Circulatory
5. Device
6. Endocrine/metabolic
7. ENT (ear, nose, throat)
8. Eyes
9. Haematological
10. Hepatobiliary
11. Immunological
12. Infections
13. Lactation exposure
14. Musculoskeletal
15. Neoplasms
16. Neurological
17. Poisoning
18. Pregnancy exposure
19. Psychiatric
20. Respiratory
21. Skin
22. Surgery
23. Unclassified
24. Urogenital

[1] Intensive Medicines Monitoring Programme.

Annex 4. Clinical Category Eyes, IMMP[1] events dictionary

Eyes System Organ Class IMMP Events Dictionary

EYES	Non-specific		Eye pain	10.000
EYES	Non-specific		Eyes irritable	10.020
EYES	Non-specific		Eyes tired	10.070
EYES	Non-specific		Hyperaemia	10.100
EYES	Non-specific		Red eyes	10.100
EYES	Non-specific		Bulging eyes	10.200
EYES	Visual	Acuity	Blindness	20.000
EYES	Visual	Acuity	Blindness temporary	20.005
EYES	Visual	Acuity	Amaurosis fugax	20.010
EYES	Visual	Acuity	Blurred vision	20.100
EYES	Visual	Acuity	Blurred vision, episodic	20.102
EYES	Visual	Acuity	Blurred vision, transient	20.103
EYES	Visual	Acuity	Blurred vision, worse	20.104
EYES	Visual	Acuity	Vision reduced	20.105
EYES	Visual	Acuity	Tunnel vision	20.108
EYES	Visual	Acuity	Vision abnormal	20.110
EYES	Visual	Acuity	Accommodation abnormal	20.150
EYES	Visual	Acuity	Scotoma	20.000
EYES	Visual	Acuity	Visual field defect	20.210
EYES	Visual	Disturbance	Visual trails	20.300
EYES	Visual	Disturbance	Ghosting	20.310
EYES	Visual	Disturbance	Flashing	20.320
EYES	Visual	Disturbance	Teichopsia	20.330
EYES	Visual	Disturbance	Chromastopsia	20.400
EYES	Visual	Disturbance	Photophobia	20.600
EYES	Intraocular	Retinal	Retinal detachment	30.000
EYES	Intraocular	Retinal	Angioid streaks retina	30.100
EYES	Intraocular	Retinal	Retinopathy	30.210
EYES	Intraocular	Retinal	Retinopathy, diabetic	30.215
EYES	Intraocular	Retinal	Retinitis	30.250
EYES	Intraocular	Retinal	Macular degeneration	30.300
EYES	Intraocular	Vascular	Optic neuropathy ischaemic	30.500
EYES	Intraocular	Vascular	Occlusion macular artery	30.510
EYES	Intraocular	Vascular	Retinal haemorrhage	30.520
EYES	Intraocular	Vitreous	Vitreous detachment	30.600
EYES	Intraocular	Gliosis	Gliosis preretinal	30.800
EYES	Intraocular	Lens	Cataract	40.000
EYES	Intraocular	Lens	Cataract, worse	40.010
EYES	Intraocular	Pressure	Glaucoma	50.000
EYES	Intraocular	Pressure	Glaucoma, acute	50.050
EYES	Intraocular	Uveal tract	Iritis	60.000
EYES	Intraocular	Uveal tract	Uveitis anterior	60.010
EYES	Intraocular	Uveal tract	Uveitis posterior	60.020
EYES	Intraocular	Pupillary	Mydriasis	61.000
EYES	Intraocular	Pupillary	Miosis	61.010
EYES	Intraocular	Pupillary	Anisocoria	61.050
EYES	Corneal	Opacity	Corneal deposits	70.000
EYES	Corneal	Opacity	Corneal infiltration	70.100
EYES	Corneal	Inflammation	Keratitis	70.200
EYES	Corneal	Inflammation	Corneal ulcer	70.300
EYES	Corneal	Anatomical	Keratoconus	70.400
EYES	Corneal	Infection	Herpes ophthalmicus	70.500
EYES	Conjunctival	Infection	Conjunctivitis	75.000
EYES	Conjunctival	Inflammatory	Episcleritis	75.100
EYES	Conjunctival	Allergy	Conjunctivitis allergic	75.100
EYES	Conjunctival	Haemorrhage	Subconjunctival harmorrhage	75.200
EYES	Tear secretion	Reduced	Xerophthalmia	76.000
EYES	Tear secretion	Reduced	Dry eyes	76.000
EYES	Tear secretion	Increased	Epiphora	76.200
EYES	Eyelid	Infection	Blepharitis	80.100
EYES	Eyelid	Infection	Stye	80.150
EYES	Eyelid	Infection	Meibomiam cyst	80.160
EYES	Eyelid	Anatomical	Ectropion	80.500
EYES	Eyelid	Anatomical	Entropion	80.550
EYES	Eyelid	Anatomical	Pterygium	80.800

[1] Intensive Medicines Monitoring Programme.

Annex 5. Events collation, Circulatory, omeprazole –IMMP[1] sample listing

Omeprazole

Event	Sex	Age	Dose Mcg/d	Dur	Rel	Report No.
Circulatory cont...						
CHF, worse	F	82	40	23 m	4	R29103 (D)
CHF, worse	F	71	20		4	F32350 (D)
CHF, worse	F	79	20	1 d	4	F35486 (D)
CHF, worse	M	82	20	18 m	4	S33587
CHF, worse	M	71	20		4	FI/1681 (D)
CHF, worse	M	70	20		4	PI/1009
CHF, worse	M		20	15 m	4	SI/2170 (D)
CHF, worse	F		40	2 y	4	SI/2066 (D)
CHF, worse	F		20	1 y	4	SI/2187
CHF, worse	F	77	20	8 m	4	FI/2355
LVF	M	85		16 m	4	S34292 (D)
LVF	M	61	20	6 w	4	F31854
LVF	M	68	20	2 y	4	S33920 (D)
LVF	M	49	40		4	S33779 (D)
LVF	M	83	20		4	FI/1884 (D)
LVF	M	78	20		4	FI/1907
LVF	M	76	20	14 m	4	FI/2699 (D)
Dyspnoea	F		20	10 m	4	FI/2309
Oedema	F		20		3	R29310
Oedema	F		20	1 d	2	R22484 *
Oedema	F	78	20	2 y	3	F31247
Oedema	F	81	20	4 y	4	S32689
Oedema	F		20		4	RI/1632
Oedema	M	79	20		4	PI/1747
Oedema	M	93	40	20 m	4	PI/2150
Oedema (nifedipine)	F	77	20		3	F26855
Cardiomyopathy	F		40		4	S33784 (D)
Cardiac disease unspecified	M	73	40		4	FI/1867 (D)
Cardiac disease unspecified	F	73	40		4	FI/1190 (D)
Angina	F	82	40	14 m	4	FI/2002
Angina	M	78	40	18 m	4	FI/2168
Angina, unstable	M	71	20		4	P30321
Angina, unstable	F	80	20	2 w	4	F 33463
Angina, unstable	M	46	40		4	FI/1456
Angina, unstable	F	74	20	3 m	4	SI/2559
Angina, unstable	M	68	40	3 y	4	SI/2561 *
Angina, unstable	F	66	40	9 m	4	FI/2578
Angina, worse	F	63	20	12 m	4	S38616
Angina, worse	M	68	40		4	RI/1955
Angina, worse	M		20		4	FI/1604
Ischaemic heart disease	M	67	20		4	CI/167 (D)
Ischaemic heart disease	M	74	20	21 m	4	SI/2125 (D)
Ischaemic heart disease, worse	F	82	20		4	FI/22395
Chest pain	F	52	20	14 m	4	S32690
Chest pain	M	71	20	3 y	4	F34342
Chest pain	F	72	20		4	FI/1575
Chest tightness (sumatriptan)	F	47	20	1 w	4	R29616
Chest tightness (sumatriptan)	F	50	20	13 m	3	R31724
Myocardial infarction	M	76	40	2 y	4	R30286 (D)
Myocardial infarction	M		20	6 w	4	C30921 (D)
Myocardial infarction	F	84	20		4	F33406 (D)
Myocardial infarction	F	78	20	2 y	3	S34995 (D)
Myocardial infarction	M	70	20	13 m	4	F32539 (D)
Myocardial infarction	F	89	20	4 y	4	F36441 (D)

[1] Intensive Medicines Monitoring Programme.

Annex 6. Comparative events profiles (celecoxib and rofecoxib) – IMMP[1] sample listing

Figure 1: Profile of events for celexocix (n=1714) and rofecoxib (n=982)

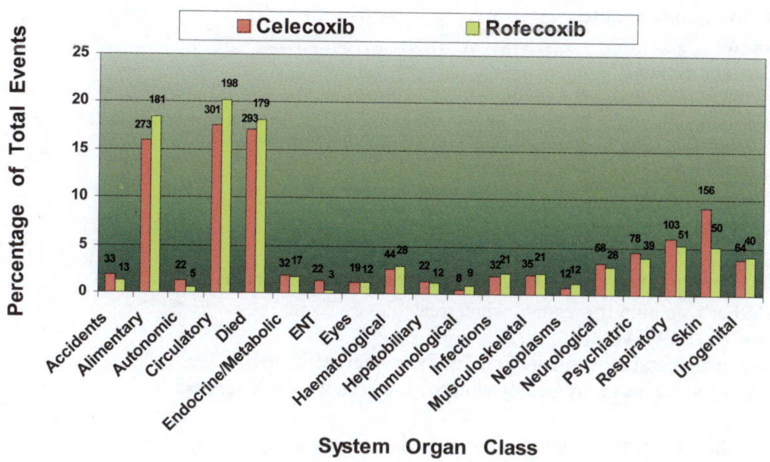

1 Intensive Medicines Monitoring Programme.

Annex 7A. Pregnancy enquiry questionnaire

(for all women aged 14–50 years of age not known to be pregnant at the time of ACT treatment. Follow-up four months after treatment)

Health worker: ………………………… Date of interview…../…../……

A. Woman's details:
Name: …………………………………………………
Contact details:
……………………………………………………………………………
Date of birth: …./…./….   **or**   Age ……………(known or estimated)
Date of treatment with monitored antimalarial: ……./……/…….
Health facility where treated: ………………………..
Treatment facility number (if available): …………………..
No history of pregnancy: □

B. If pregnant, estimate stage of pregnancy at exposure to antimalarial
Mother's opinion if pregnant when treated: yes □; no □
Date of LMP if known: …../…./……
Date when fetal movements first felt by mother (estimated): ……/……/…….
Estimated weeks of pregnancy at current interview: ……….weeks

Has she attended an antenatal clinic for this pregnancy? yes □; no □
Name of clinic she has attended or will attend …………………………………………
Clinic Number (if available)……………

At what stage was she exposed to the antimalarial(s)? (*Tick all if applicable, or as many as necessary, if several treatments have been given*)
1st trimester □; 2nd trimester □; 3rd trimester □; at term □

C. Any abnormalities of pregnancy?
Abnormalities of pregnancy: None □   Don't know □
Miscarriage □ date:……/……/……..   Therapeutic abortion □

Date	Description of pregnancy abnormalities

Baby not yet born □ Baby already born □; Date of birth ……/……/…….
If woman is pregnant, arrange follow-up using the Pregnancy **Progress** Questionnaire
If baby has been born, please complete the Pregnancy **Outcome** Questionnaire

Please return this questionnaire to the Pharmacovigilance Centre according to local procedure

Annex 7B. Pregnancy Progress Questionnaire

(for all women who were pregnant when treated with the antimalarial(s) being monitored)

Attempt to complete a Pregnancy Progress Questionnaire each time she attends an antenatal clinic.

Health worker: ………………………… Date of interview…../…../……

A. Woman's details:

Name: …………………………………………………

Contact details: ……………………………………………………………

Date of birth: …./…./…. **or** Age ……………(known or estimated)

Name of clinic ……………………………………………

Clinic number ………………

Estimated weeks of pregnancy at current examination: ……….weeks

B. Medicines given

Please record medicines given since last visit and at this visit

Date	Medicine	Dose schedule	Reason

C. Any abnormalities of pregnancy?

Abnormalities of pregnancy: None identified □

Miscarriage □ date:……/……/…….. Therapeutic abortion □

Date	Description of pregnancy abnormalities

Baby not yet born □ Baby already born □; date of birth ……/……/…….

If baby has been born, please complete the Pregnancy *Outcome* Questionnaire

Please return this questionnaire to the Pharmacovigilance Centre according to local procedure

Annex 7C. Pregnancy Outcome Questionnaire

Treatment centre/Clinic: …………………………….
Contact person: ………………………….

A. Woman's details:

Name: …………………………………………………
Clinic Number……………
Contact details: ………………………………………………………………………….

Date of birth: …./…./….
Does she think she was pregnant when treated with the antimalarial? yes □; no □

B. Stage of pregnancy at exposure

LMP if known: …../…./…… Estimated weeks of pregnancy at current examination: ……….weeks

At what stage was she exposed to the antimalarials? (*Tick all if applicable, or as many as necessary*)

1st trimester □; 2nd trimester □; 3rd trimester □; At term □

C. Outcome of pregnancy

Date of birth ……/……/…. Not yet born □
1. Abnormalities of pregnancy: None □ Don't know □ Miscarriage □
date:……/……/…….. Therapeutic abortion □

Date	Description of pregnancy abnormalities

2. Abnormalities of labour (*describe below*) None □; Don't know □
Date of delivery: ……./……./……..

3. Abnormalities of foetus or infant Don't know □ Fetal death □ date …../…../……
None identified at birth □; None identified at 3 months □; None identified at 1 year □

Date identified	Description of any abnormalities

D. Breastfeeding

1. Did the mother breastfeed the infant while on treatment? Yes □; No □; Don't know □
2. If yes, when was the baby first exposed with the mother on treatment?
From birth □; From age …………………..; Don't know □
3. Was there any effect on the infant? Yes □; No □; Don't know □
4. If yes, please describe:

Date of follow-up……../……/……

Annex 8. Deaths (as events) with omeprazole – IMMP[1] sample listing

Omeprazole

Event	Sex	Age	Dose Mcg/d	Dur	Rel	Report No.
DIED - Circulatory cont...						
Vascular disease	F	74	20	17 m	4	SI/2814 (D)
Vascular occlusion	M	62	40	1 d	4	FI/2285 (D)
Venous thrombosis,embolism pulmonary,bronchopneumonia	M	87	20	1 y	4	F33114 (D)
Ventricular fibrillation, CHF	M	74	20	3 m	4	C33504 (D)
- Endocrine/Metabolic						
Addisons disease	M		20	2 y	4	S36594 (D)
Alcoholism	M	67	20	4 m	4	FI/2776 (D)
Alpha 1 antitrypsin deficiency	F	55	40		4	S38674 (D)
Cachexia	M	75	20	3 y	4	FI/2779 (D)
Debility	F	78	20	2 y	4	FI/2945 (D)
Dehydration	M	75	20	3 y	4	FI/2399 (D)
Dehydration, renal failure	F	81	20	17 m	4	SI/2443 (D)
Diabetes mellitus	M	88	20	16 m	4	S34537 (D)
- Haematological						
Aplastic anaemia	F	86	20	18 m	3	S28676 (D)
Aplastic anaemia (leukemia)	F	24	40	3 m	4	FI/2373 (D)
Bleeding disorder, renal failure	F		20	2 y	4	S27986 (D)
Bleeding, bowel	F	86	20	16 m	4	C32989 (D)
Leukemia	M	80	20	10 m	4	F33027 (D)
Leukemia	M	28	20		5	CI/1165 (D)
Leukemia, acute myeloid	F	54		1 w	4	FI/1227 (D)
Macroglobulinaemia	M	68	20	1 w	4	CI/2032 (D)
Myelodysplasia	F	68	40	4 m	4	F32540 (D)
Myelodysplastic syndrome	F	93	20	2 y	4	SI/2606 (D)
Myelodysplastic syndrome, pulmonary fibrosis	F	81	40		4	CI/1271 (D)
Myeloproliferative disorder	M	83	20	2 m	4	FI/2810 (D)
- Hepatobiliary						
Biliary cirrhosis	F	66	40	20 m	4	FI/2812 (D)
Hepatic cirrhosis	M	74	20	18 m	4	S33223 (D)
Hepatic cirrhosis	F	76	20		4	CI/2383 (D)
Hepatic cirrhosis	M	60	40		4	CI/2408 (D)
Hepatic failure	M	77	40	1 m	4	FI/5654 (D)
Hepatic failure	M	62	20	5 m	4	FI/2863 (D)
Hepatic failure (azathioprine)	M	31	20		4	RI/1587 (D)
Liver disease alcoholic	M	66	40	2 y	4	S33689 (D)
- Immunological						
AIDS	M	40	20	4 m	4	FI/2305 (D)
Myocarditis, MI	F	78	20	2 y	3	S30915 (D)

[1] Intensive Medicines Monitoring Programme.

Annex 9. Eye events listing from IMMP[1]

Collation of events for SOC Eyes COX-2 inhibitors

Demonstration of signal

EYES

Event	Code	Sex	Age	Drug	Dose	Dur	Rel	Report No.
Non Specific								
Eye pain	10.000	M	59	CEL	200	6 d	1	R52816*
Eye pain	10.000	F	71	CEL	200	738 d	4	F53137
Eye pain	10.000	M		CEL	200	287 d	4	F60469*
Eye pain	10.000	F	52	CEL	100	835 d	4	F60564
Eyes irritable	10.020	M	70	CEL	400		4	F56205
Eyes irritable	10.020	F	67	CEL	100	785 d	4	F62704
Eyes irritable	10.020	M	71	ROF			4	F58175
Eyes irritable	10.020	F	64	ROF	12.5	447 d	4	F69660
Red eyes	10.100	M		CEL	200	287 d	4	F60069*
Red eyes	10.100	M	54	ROF	25	143 d	4	F60155
Dry eyes	10.300	F	64	CEL	100	620 d	4	F62269
Visual								
Acuity								
Blurred vision	20.100	F	53	CEL	200	4 m	2	R46379*
Blurred vision	20.100	F	59	CEL	200	7 w	2	A47419*
Blurred vision	20.100	F	79	CEL	200	4 m	3	F54575
Blurred vision	20.100	F	71	CEL	200	392 d	4	F56537
Blurred vision	20.100	F	41	VAD		1 d	3	R59759*
Blurred vision (atenolol)	20.100	M	58	ROF		10 d	3	R478404*
Blurred vision (cilazapril)	20.100	F	81	ETO	60	42 d	2	A56946*
Vision abnormal	20.100	F	71	CEL	200		2	F50058*
Vision abnormal	20.100	F	73	CEL	200		2	R52142*
Vision abnormal	20.100	M	45	CEL	200	76 d	3	F52120
Vision abnormal	20.100	M	86	ETO	120	21 d	2	F60305*
Vision reduced	20.200	F	81	CEL	200	27 d	2	B46049*
Vision reduced	20.200	F	74	CEL	200		3	P55508
Vision reduced	20.200	F	78	ETO	60	1 d	2	R607460*
Vision reduced	20.200	M	78	ROF	50	1 d	2	R50797*
Vision reduced	20.200	F	88	ROF	25		2	F57153*
Visual field defect	20.220	M	81	CEL	100	3 w	1	R50269*
Visual field defect	20.220	M	61	ROF	25	26 d	2	F53280*
Blindness temporary	20.310	M	78	ROF	50	1d	2	F58471*
Disturbance								
Flashing	20.500	M	77	CEL	200	8 m	4	F53547
Flashing	20.500	F	78	CEL	200	188 d	4	F59624*
Teichopsia	20.550	F	72	ETO	60	184 d	3	F61676
Teichopsia	20.550	M	77	ROF	12.5		2	B47874*
Teichopsia	20.550	F	73	ROF	12.5	2 d	2	A56985*
Intraocular								
Retinal haemorrhage	30.100	M	84	ROF	25	15 w	4	F53051
Vitreous detachment	35.000	F	65	CEL	100	869 d	4	F59161
Vitreous detachment	35.000	F	65	ROF	12.5	8 m	4	F53246
Cataract	40.000	F	78	CEL	200	46 d	4	F59324*
Cataract, worse	40.000	F	84	CEL	200		4	F57441
Glaucoma	50.000	M	74	CEL	200		3	F59252*
Uveitis posterior	60.010	F	67	CEL	200		4	F54603
Corneal								
Keratitis	70.200	M	46	CEL	299	640 d	4	F58745
Keratitis	70.200	F	70	ROF	12.5		4	F54854*
Conjunctival								
Infection								
Conjunctivitis	80.000	F	61	CEL	200		4	F54944
Conjunctivitis	80.000	F	77	CEL	200	49 d	4	F50177*
Conjunctivitis	80.000	F	53	CEL	200	8 d	4	F57163
Conjunctivitis	80.000	F	42	CEL	200	113 d	4	F52138
Conjunctivitis	80.000	F	56	CEL	400	27 m	4	F53139
Conjunctivitis	80.000	F	76	CEL	100	46 d	4	F59424
Conjunctivitis	80.000	F	53	CEL	100	890 d	4	P559550
Conjunctivitis	80.000	F	55	ROF	50		1	R56688*

Allergy								
Conjunctivitis allergic	80.050	M	43	CEL	200	1 w	3	B43081*
Conjunctivitis allergic	80.050	F	46	ROF	25	4 m	4	F59972
Haemorrhage								
Subconjunctival haemorrhage	80.200	M	68	CEL	400	531 d	4	F58012
Subconjunctival haemorrhage	80.200	F	83	CEL	100	12 d	4	F60120
Subconjunctival haemorrhage (azathioprine, prednisone)	80.200	F	68	ROF	25	307 d	3	F56344
Eyelid								
Blepharitis	80.300	F	59	CEL	700	5 m	4	F54489
Meibomian cyst	80.360	F	54	CEL	200	6 m	4	F57543

[1] Intensive Medicines Monitoring Programme.

Annex 10. Drug–drug associations with celecoxib – IMMP[1] sample listing

Event	Sex	Age	Dose Mg/d	Dur	Rel	Report No.
ASSOCIATIONS 46 6.73 %						
Alendronate, gastric ulcer bleeding, anaemia	F	89	100	1 m	3	R 49222 *
Allopurinol, duodenal ulcer, oesophagitis	M	52	200		4	B 46665 *
Allopurinol, renal failure acute	F	71	200		3	R 47848 *
Amiodarone, dyspnoea	F	79	400	7 d	2	R 48563 *
Amitriptyline, hypertension, hemianopia	F	80			3	B 42818
Amitriptyline, myocardial infarction	F	80	200	5 d	3	R 43633 *
Amitriptyline, tachycardia	F	45	200	3 d	3	R 44655 *
Aspirin, duodenal ulcer bleeding	F	82	100	2 m	3	B 45376 *
Aspirin, gastric ulcer bleeding	F	70	200	5 m	3	F 50693 *
Aspirin, gastric ulcer bleeding, anaemia	F	89	100	1 m	2	R 48722 *
Aspirin, haematemesis, melena, duodenal ulcer	M	72	200	3 w	3	B 47881 *
Aspirin, melena, myocardial infarction	M	71			3	D 48943 *
Bendrofluazide, dyspnoea, weakness	F	84		19 m	2	R 51808 *
Bupropion, anxiety, insomnia	F	64	100	1 m	4	D 41552
Cilazapril, dyspnoea, weakness	F	84		19 m	2	R 51298 *
Cisapride, vomiting, hysteria, hypokinesia	F	47	100	1 d	4	R 46338
Diclofenac, nephritis interstitial	M	73		6 w	3	R 46646 *
Hair dye, urticaria, angioedema, wheeze	F	74	200	1 h	2	B 43835 *
Hepatitis B vaccine, flushing, dizziness skin cold clammy, malaise	F	42	100	15 mi	4	R 50467
Ibuprofen, LFTs abnormal	F	61	200	1 m	3	B 47516
Leflunamide, liver injury cholestatic	F	65	200	8 m	4	R 48407 *
Leflunomide, tendon rupture, arm pain	M	48			4	R 47912
Methotrexate, liver injury cholestatic	F	65	200	14 m	4	R 47417 *
Metoprolol, angioedema	F	73	200		4	R 52124
Olanzapine, akathisia	F	69	200	16 d	4	R 50436 *
Pantoprazole, rash	F	78	100	3 d	4	R 46646
Paroxetine, hyponatraemia	F	79	200	2 d	4	R 45502 *
Perfume, anaphylactoid reaction	F	60	200		4	R 56462 *
Prednisone, chest pain	F	57	400	2 h	3	B 46877 *
Prednisone, duodenal ulcer	F	84	200	12 d	3	R 46489 *
Prednisone, haematemesis	M	55	200	4 m	3	B 44195 (D)
Prednisone, melena	F	94	400	5 d	3	R 47140 *
Prednisone, tendon rupture, arm pain	M	48			4	R 41312
Quinapril, cough, dyspnoea	M	72	200	1 w	4	R 47288 *
Quinapril, headache, dental caries, hypertension therapeutic response decreased	M	67	200	3 m	2	B 43831 *
Quinapril, urticaria, angioedema, wheeze	F	74	200		3	B 43849 *
Quinine, thrombocyotpenia, bleeding	F	53	200	7 d	3	B 44505 *
Spironolactone, hyponatraemia	F	86	100		3	F 51665 *
Sulphasalazine,bladder discomfort,rash papular,pruritus	F	68	200		4	R 47589 DR
Synvisc, pain joint	F	41	200	1 d	4	R 48246
Warfarin, INR increased	F	87	200	9 d	2	R 48931 *
Warfarin, INR increased	F	69	200	3 d	3	R 49106
Warfarin, INR increased, haematuria	M	59	400	1 d	2	B 41355 *
Warfarin, aortic aneurysm ruptured	M	78	200	6 w	4	R 48024 (D)
AUTONOMIC 14 2.05 %						
Faintness	M	42	200	3 h	3	R 46403 *
Faintness	F	64		30 mi	2	R 46444 *
Sweating	F	38			2	B 43527 *
Sweating	M	42	200	3 h	3	R 46460 *
Sweating	F	68	200	10 d	1	A 46547 *
Sweating	M	51	200	2 h	1	R 49083 *
Skin cold clammy	F	64		30 mi	2	R 46945 *
Skin cold clammy (hepatitis B vaccine)	F	42	100	3 m	4	R 50007
Shivering	M	26	200	1 h	1	R 49168 *
Fever	M	82	200	4 d	3	B 42160 *
Hot feeling	F	68	200	10 d	1	A 46536 *
Mouth dry	F	77	400	3 m	3	R 49441 *
Nasal congestion	F	54	400	2 d	3	F 52502
*Rhinorrhoea	F	56	200	1 d	1	A 51480 *

[1] Intensive Medicines Monitoring Programme.

Annex 11. A selection of helpful web sites

WHO Headquarters

A great deal of information is available here, including access to WHO publications.
http://www.who.int/en/

the Uppsala Monitoring Centre (UMC)

This site provides very useful information about practical pharmacovigilance including definitions and advice on pharmacovigilance policy.
http://www.who-umc.org/

Vigisearch

Provides access to the WHO worldwide database of adverse reactions and dictionaries Open DD-online (Drug Dictionary), Open ATC-online (ATC classification) and Open WHO-ART-online (adverse reaction terminology).
https://vigisearch.who-umc.org/login.asp

European Medicines Agency

This is a useful resource on product information, current issues and regulatory actions.
http://www.emea.europa.eu

Food and Drug Administration (FDA), USA

This is a useful resource on product information, current issues and regulatory actions.
http://www.fda.gov/

Communicable Diseases Centre, USA

This site has a lot of information and statistics on communicable diseases and medicines related to their treatment.
http://www.cdc.gov/

NZ regulatory web site

This is a good resource for data sheets for medicines and patient leaflets. It also has articles in *Prescriber Update*, many of which come from the National Centre.
http://www.medsafe.govt.nz/

Natural Standard

The best and most authoritative web site available on herbal medicines. Users are required to register and pay a fee.
http://www.naturalstandard.com/

British National Formulary

A good and reliable resource for information on medicines.

Literature resource

The WHO Health Inter-Network Access to Research Initiative (HINARI). This provides free or very low-cost online access to the major journals in biomedical and related social sciences to local, not-for-profit institutions in developing countries.
http://www.who.int/hinari/about/en/

Micromedex/Drugdex/Martindale

All are available through this web site. Users are required to register and pay a fee. This is probably the most convenient and comprehensive source of information on medicines.
https://www.thomsonhc.com/home/dispatch/PFDefaultActionId/pf.LoginAction/ssl/true

PubMed

This is a good literature resource. Abstracts are available free.
http://www.ncbi.nlm.nih.gov/entrez/query.fcgi?CMD=search&DB=pubmed

Anatomical Therapeutic Chemical (ATC) Classification and codes

The ATC classification system is maintained by the WHO Collaborating Centre for Drug Statistics Methodology
http://www.whocc.no/atcddd/

International Society of Pharmacovigilance (ISOP)

This is an important international society. Their web site gives information about meetings and training courses.
www.isoponline.org

International Society for Pharmacoepidemiology (ISPE)

This site is a useful source of information on the activities of the society and for guidelines on risk management and links to relevant information.
www.pharmacoepi.org

International Uniform Requirements for Manuscripts Submitted to Biomedical Journals

An essential resource when writing articles, this site gives guidance on structure of articles and formats for references.

http://www.icmje.org/

British Medical Journal (BMJ)

Free access to some articles is available and the table of contents for each issue can be seen.

http://bmj.bmjjournals.com/

Medline

This site gives access to a list of journal abbreviations. It is an essential resource for compiling literature references and checking the details of journals referred to in articles in the literature.

http://www.ncbi.nlm.nih.gov/entrez/query.fcgi?db=Journals&itool=toolbar

Cytochrome P450 enzymes

A listing of the enzymes with the medicines affected is provided. This is a useful resource when researching possible interactions.

http://medicine.iupui.edu/flockhart/table.htm

ICD-10

An electronic searchable version of ICD-10 is available on this web site.

http://www.who.int/classifications/apps/icd/icd10online/

Annex 12. Published resources

(See also list of selected websites Annex 11)

Safety monitoring of medicinal products: Guidelines for setting up and running a Pharmacovigilance Centre. Uppsala, Sweden, The Uppsala Monitoring Centre, 2000.

Safety of medicines: A guide to detecting and reporting adverse drug reactions. Geneva, World Health Organization, 2002.

The importance of pharmacovigilance: Safety monitoring of medicinal products. Geneva, World Health Organization, 2002.

The safety of medicines in public health programmes: Pharmacovigilance an essential tool. Geneva, World Health Organization, 2006

Coulter DM. The New Zealand Intensive Medicines Monitoring Programme in pro-active safety surveillance. *Pharmacoepidemiology and Drug Safety*, 2000, 9:273–280.

Harrison-Woolrych M, Coulter DM. PEM in New Zealand. In: Mann R, Andrews E, eds. *Pharmacovigilance*, 2nd ed. Chichester, John Wiley, 2007:317–332.

Shakir Saad AW. PEM in the UK. In: Mann R, Andrews E, eds. *Pharmacovigilance*, 2nd ed. Chichester, John Wiley, 2007.

Coulter DM. Signal generation in the New Zealand Intensive Medicines Monitoring Programme. *Drug Safety*, 2002, 25:433–439.

Coulter DM. Privacy issues and the monitoring of sumatriptan in the NZ IMMP. *Pharmacoepidemiology and Drug Safety*, 2001, 10:663–667.

Reporting Adverse Drug reactions: Definitions of Terms and Criteria for their use. Geneva, Council for International Organizations of Medical Sciences (CIOMS), 1999.

Annex 13. Contacts

WHO Headquarters, Geneva

Dr Mary Couper
Medical Officer
Telephone +41 22 791 3643
Email: couperm@who.int

Dr Shanthi Pal
Technical Officer
Telephone +41 22 7911318
Email: pals@who.int

Quality Assurance and Safety Medicines
World Health Organization
20, Avenue Appia
CH-1211 Geneva 27
Switzerland

Dr Andrea Bosman
Medical Officer
Telephone +41 22 791 3860
Email: bosmana@who.int

Global Malaria Programme
World Health Organization
20, Avenue Appia
CH-1211 Geneva 27
Switzerland

The Uppsala Monitoring Centre (WHO Collaborating Centre)

Professor I.R Edwards
Director
WHO Collaborating Centre for International Drug Monitoring
Email: ralph.edwards@who-umc.org

Mr Sten Olsson
Manager External Affairs
WHO Collaborating Centre for International Drug Monitoring
Email: sten.olsson@who-umc.org

For advice on Cohort Event Monitoring

Associate Professor David Coulter
Dunedin 9010
New Zealand
Telephone +64 3 477 4269
Email: dmcoulter@xtra.co.nz

For advice on communication

Mr Bruce Hugman
Chiang Rai – 57000 – Thailand
Phone/fax: +66 53 750876
Mobile: +66 89 6 35 35 94
Email: mail@brucehugman.net
Website: www.brucehugman.net

Annex 14. The importance of communication

Throughout this manual, effective communication has been emphasized as an essential part of good pharmacovigilance. This Annex gives a brief overview of some of the most important knowledge and skills in communication, without which even the best system will not fulfil its potential.

Know your audience

It is critical to tailor all your materials and activities closely to the abilities and preferences of your many audiences. These days, even very serious people have little time or short attention spans especially for printed materials, and everything needs to be as brief, clear and persuasive as possible. Not everyone will share your priorities and values, so it's important to know the state of mind of your recipients so that the message really does get under their skin. Remember that within just one audience (pharmacists, for example) there will be a very wide range of ability, literacy, motivation and so on. Get to know your audiences through direct engagement and exchange with them: such knowledge will pay dividends.

Seek feedback

One of the best ways to understand your audiences is to actively seek feedback from them about your materials and what you are doing. Always pilot-test a project like the production of a reporting form or a new explanatory leaflet: find out what a range of recipients think about your work and then modify the content and the approach in the light of their views. Those of us working at desks in centralized offices often misjudge our recipients and so our messages don't get the attention they deserve.

Give feedback and provide benefits

To stimulate collaboration and motivate colleagues, there needs to be some real benefit to be gained from making the effort to report ADRs, or to monitor public health programmes, or take part in other activities. At the lowest level, appreciation (a "pat on the back") is a powerful motivator, but feedback about how information has helped improve patient safety, or a special newsletter for reporters and collaborators, or any other acceptable incentive will make a difference. There are still too many systems in which doctors, nurses and pharmacists are expected to help, but get no acknowledgement or feedback at all. We cannot simply rely on everyone being selfless, dedicated altruists.

Make your communications stand out

The competition for everyone's attention at every moment of the day is extreme, and health care professionals, the world over, are buried in printed materials of all kinds – many of them attractive, impressive and influential, but they are often put in the bin without so much as a glance.

We need to be sure that our materials look attractive and professional and, as far as possible, irresistible! Reporting forms need to look engaging and inviting, not merely produced amateurishly on a word processor in black and white. Some input from a graphic designer will make all the difference to the quality (and success) of forms and every piece of printed or electronic material. There may be a small initial cost, but this will be offset by the reduction in numbers of forms wasted and thrown away, and in increased interest and involvement. We are *competing* for people's attention, and need to take that challenge seriously. (Just look in any decent magazine and see how elegantly and powerfully commercial messages are promoted.)

Writing style

Writing is another of those advanced skills which every pharmacovigilance professional is expected to be born with. Good writing is hard work and essential for effective communication. Try to use people whose writing skills are advanced already, but if there is no such person, follow these rules:

- Write in the simplest, clearest language suitable for the task.
- Get your main points over at the beginning, and repeat them at the end.
- Keep sentences and paragraphs short.
- Use subheadings and bullet points as much as you can.
- When there is a lot of subsidiary or supporting material, try to separate it from the main message content.
- Read your writing aloud to see how it sounds – this is one of the best tests possible.
- Get some members of your intended audience to read and comment on what you have written.

Repeat the message

Remember that in the hurly-burly of workaday life, many people will miss a message which is sent only once. *One communication is no communication.* Repeat your message again and again, in different forms and through different channels, until you know that people have received it and are being influenced by it – and this might take years rather than months. Changing people's attitudes, values and behaviour takes an immense amount of time and effort.

Get personal

The closer your communications get to being one-to-one and face-to-face, the more effective they will be. A mailing of a thousand leaflets will have far less effect than ten mailings of ten leaflets carefully tailored to subgroups of the audience. And, of course, mailings will have far less effect than meeting people in small groups or individually. Within the limits of your budget and resources, get as close to your recipients as you can.

Journalists

The media in all its forms can become a powerful ally of health care and patient safety if journalists are dealt with personally and professionally. Most bad press comes from alienated journalists who have never been contacted, briefed or educated in the complexities of medicine. Get some training in media relations; meet some of your local editors and health journalists; explore what you can achieve together. Suspicion and avoidance simply generate more suspicion and hostility. (The UMC publication *Dialogue in Pharmacovigilance* contains guidance on media relations, and there are lots of books and useful websites.) And – never say, "No comment".

Meetings

Meetings are the form of group communication which probably cause more anxiety and frustration, and waste more time than any other single activity. While they are sometimes productive, they are often depressing and demoralizing. Meetings can be well-run, short, effective and uplifting. Running effective meetings requires a very specific set of knowledge and skills which can be learnt by anyone keen enough to reduce the hours of their own and other people's lives wasted sitting pointlessly in meeting-rooms. Again, there are lots of good books and websites which will reveal how staff meetings, seminars, conferences and consultations can be made stimulating and productive.

The message

The safety of patients worldwide is served by dedicated professionals doing their work well, but that work will never reach its considerable potential without excellent supporting communications. Excellent communications require a degree of expertise, creativity and skill which not all officials and scientists have as a matter of course. In every organization there is likely to be someone with a communications gift: look for them and use them if you can; otherwise put communications on your regular agenda as a high priority and give the activity of communicating as much attention as the content of what you wish to communicate.

[Contributed by Bruce Hugman

mail@brucehugman.net]

Annex 15. Power and sample size analysis for statistical comparison of an event in two cohorts

Table 1 With an incidence of the event of 0.1% in one cohort

*Significance level**	*Power#*	*Incidence of ADE in one therapy*	*RR*	*Sample Size (each group)*
0.05	0.80	0.10%	2.0	25 476
0.01	0.80	0.10%	2.0	36 961
0.05	0.80	0.10%	3.0	8805
0.01	0.80	0.10%	3.0	12 636
0.05	0.80	0.10%	4.0	4993
0.01	0.80	0.10%	4.0	7123
0.05	0.80	0.10%	5.0	3416
0.01	0.80	0.10%	5.0	4853
0.05	0.80	0.10%	6.0	2573
0.01	0.80	0.10%	6.0	3647
0.05	0.65	0.10%	6.0	1913

*Significance level or α, is the type I error rate, which is the probability of falsely rejecting the null hypothesis that there was no association (in other words, RR=1) between the event of interest and the exposure therapy.
#Power, is the probability that we reject the null hypothesis correctly.

Notes:

With a sample of about 2000 patients in each therapy, the power to identify a difference in ADE rate between the two therapies would be only about 65%, even with a RR of 6.0 and 95% confidence.

Table 2 With an incidence of the event of 1.0% in one cohort

*Significance level**	*Power#*	*Incidence of ADE in one therapy*	*RR*	*Sample Size (each group)*
0.05	**0.81**	**1.0%**	**2.40**	**1500**
0.05	0.85	1.0%	2.50	1500
0.05	0.89	1.0%	2.60	1500
0.05	0.91	1.0%	2.70	1500
0.05	0.94	1.0%	2.80	1500
0.05	**0.80**	**1.0%**	**1.90**	**3000**
0.05	0.84	1.0%	1.95	3000
0.05	0.87	1.0%	2.00	3000
0.05	0.90	1.0%	2.05	3000
0.05	0.92	1.0%	2.10	3000
0.05	**0.81**	**1.0%**	**1.67**	**5000**
0.05	0.84	1.0%	1.70	5000
0.05	0.86	1.0%	1.73	5000
0.05	0.89	1.0%	1.76	5000
0.05	0.91	1.0%	1.80	5000
0.05	**0.81**	**1.0%**	**1.45**	**10 000**
0.05	0.84	1.0%	1.47	10 000
0.05	0.86	1.0%	1.49	10 000
0.05	0.90	1.0%	1.52	10 000
0.05	0.92	1.0%	1.54	10 000

*Significance level or α, is the type I error rate, which is the probability of falsely rejecting the null hypothesis that there was no association (in other words, RR=1) between the event of interest and the exposure therapy. #Power, is the probability that we reject the null hypothesis correctly.

Figure 1 Power curve of a sample size of 1500 (in each group) at incidence rates of 1.0% and 0.5% (P_0) in the control group

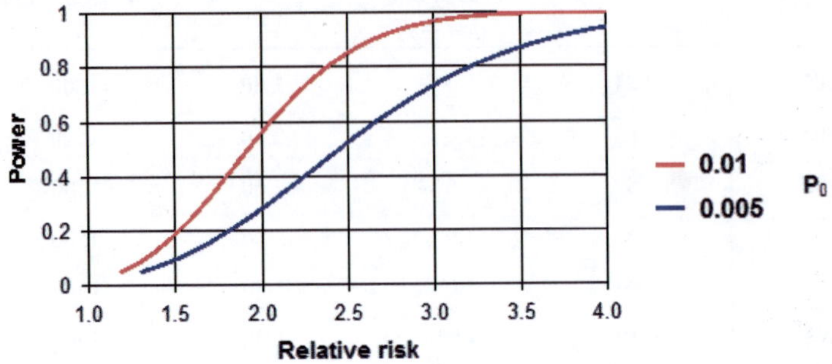

Notes:

With a sample of about 1500 in each therapy, the power to identify a significant difference in ADE rate between the two therapies would be about 81%, if the RR is 2.40 and there is a confidence of 95% (the ADE incidence rate, $\mathbf{P_0}$, is assumed to be 1.0%).

If $\mathbf{P_0}$ is 0.5%, the RR has to be more than 3.20 to reach a power of about 80% with the same sample size, as is shown in the graph above.

Tables prepared by Dr Lifeng Zhou, NZ Pharmacovigilance Centre, Department of Preventive and Social Medicine, University of Otago, Dunedin, New Zealand